THE DISTURBED CHILD

Recognition and Psychoeducational Therapy in the Classroom

The Disturbed Child

Recognition and Psychoeducational
Therapy in the Classroom

Pearl H. Berkowitz

AND

Esther P. Rothman

NEW YORK UNIVERSITY PRESS · 1960

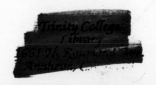

© 1960 by New York University
Library of Congress Catalog Card Number: 60–6418
Manufactured in the United States of America
By Arrangement with Washington Square Press, Inc.

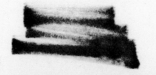

To WANDA G. WRIGHT
*Leader in the Education of the Disturbed Child,
from Whom We Learned*

Contents

CONTENTS

THE DISTURBED CHILD

Recognition and Psychoeducational Therapy in the Classroom

Chapter I

The Need for Recognizing
the Disturbed Child

The past fifty years have seen a rapidly growing interest in the psychopathology of childhood. Concepts unique to child psychopathology have evolved, based upon recognition that the principles of adult psychology cannot be applied directly to the psychology of childhood. Clarifying this concept, Mahler, Ross and DeFries [1] suggest that while the adult personality is structured before the onset of mental illness, the psychotic process in the growing child must be considered in relation to his present stage of development and cannot be equated to similar psychopathology in the adult.

It is usually easier to recognize psychological disturbances in adults than in children. Adults have had a longer life span in which to experience emotional disturbance and have generally been exposed to more involved life traumas than children. Their disturbances, therefore, are more easily discernible. The detection of disturbance in adults is also made easier by the structure of society, which puts more restrictions on adult behavior than on the behavior of children. Within the framework of most civilized societies, children are much more easily forgiven their trespasses and their peculiarities than are adults. The

---

[1] M. S. Mahler, J. R. Ross, Jr., and Z. DeFries, "Clinical Studies in Benign and Malignant Cases of Childhood Psychosis," *American Journal of Orthopsychiatry*, XIX (1949), 295–305.

unacceptable behavior of disturbed children is often tolerated because children are expected to "grow out" of these unacceptable patterns. Frequently, misbehavior on the part of children is even considered by their elders to be "cute," "smart," or "precocious," or else the child is considered just "spoiled." It happens, therefore, that deviant behavior goes unrecognized as a symptom of maladjustment. This phenomenon becomes apparent when, for example, a so-called normal child suddenly breaks away from this "normalcy" and indulges in unprovoked violence. "He was always such a good boy," a grieved parent may say, or, "I just don't understand it; he was always so quiet. He never talked back." Upon investigation it is found that although this child had functioned more or less adequately within the usual confines of society, there was much evidence of maladjustment which went unrecognized until catastrophe focused attention upon it. If a disturbance can be so subtly disguised that it goes undetected in the normal course of a child's life, the trained observer must become aware of behavior which seems to fall into the category of normalcy but which is actually symptomatic of maladjustment.

Since children spend such a large portion of their time attending school, teachers are in a unique position to observe their behavior. Teachers, armed with an objectivity that no parent can be expected to possess, are in an enviable position to study the behavior of all children. It is through such observation that maladjustment can often be detected early in childhood.

Although the teacher is not primarily a diagnostician and may not be interested in making fine classical distinctions between various types of disturbed behavior, the teacher is concerned with recognizing emotional disturbance. In the ordinary classroom, the teacher is frequently able to help the child who is emotionally disturbed by providing him with a therapeutic situation within the confines of the schoolroom. Frequently, however, children have to be referred for more intensive treatment. In either case, if the teacher is aware of the nature of the maladjustment and the behavioral patterns with which it manifests itself, the child can be helped with greater alacrity. Teachers can be alerted to the various ways in which disturbance manifests itself in the classroom so that children who need help may be given assistance either by the teacher directly or by competent professionals. Since disturbance can usually be most easily identified by observing the behavior of the child, observation is the first and simplest step in aiding those children who are seriously maladjusted. Sensitive observation permits the teacher to recognize disturbed behavior even though it may be indirectly expressed. Thus, the role of the teacher constantly enlarges itself. In addition to academic teaching, the teacher must observe behavior and be familiar with norms of psychological and emotional development as well as with its deviations.

A recent research project undertaken by the authors of this book included the collection of anecdotal and discipline records kept by teachers in the New York City schools. Many of these records indicated that the children to which they referred were considered problems of discipline by the teacher. The record was kept primarily for the purpose of obtaining disciplinary action. It is evident from the material, however, that most of the behavior described by the teachers was consistent with poor adjustment. It should have been collated for the purpose of obtaining psychological aid for these children rather than as a basis for disciplinary action. The children who were referred in this way to the school authorities were subsequently given psychological tests. The tests gave conclusive evidence that these children were really maladjusted.

In addition, this same project asked teachers to keep records on those children who were the most quiet in the classroom and who gave them the least trouble. Psychological tests were administered to these children as well. Many of these quiet, conforming children also gave indication of severe emotional conflict. The following material consists of excerpts from the records of the teachers as well as from the psychological reports.

Dorothy L.: Age 13, no discipline problem;
considered well adjusted by the teacher

ENGLISH TEACHER
"Quiet and attentive in class. Does homework faithfully, but still seems incapable of doing good work."

SCIENCE TEACHER
"She is my secretary. She is a very nice girl, but slow. She is well behaved, but does not volunteer."

MATHEMATICS TEACHER

"She is more quiet than most children, and very well mannered."

PSYCHOLOGICAL REPORT

"Dorothy is a disturbed girl who is overcome by intense anxiety and who feels that she, as well as the world, is falling apart. She tends to defend against this anxiety by denying it. Although she was obviously anxious, she consistently denied it.

"She is capable of functioning intellectually and with adequate judgment even though she is tremendously hindered by emotional instability. On the Stanford-Binet she obtained an IQ of 108, which places her in the normal range of intellectual capacity. There were indications that she is able to function at a higher level, but that she is inhibited and blocked by difficulties of emotional origin.

"Throughout the testing, Dorothy gives evidences of poor judgment and poor integrative intellectual thinking when she is confronted with emotionally charged situations. At these times, she completely falls apart and is immobilized by her anxiety. She is deeply responsive to the environment, but because she fears it so, and because her feelings of falling apart are so great, she cannot respond to the environment except in a crude, undifferentiated way. Her anxiety, however, does not prevent her from responding to environmental stimuli which are not too threatening to her. She is able to cling to the concrete elements in the environment and to control this anxiety so that she can function in the environment. Thus, she tries to concretize her experiences by reacting to the minute and unimportant details of a situation rather than to the total situation at hand. She shows evidences of forming obsessive-compulsive defenses in this attempt to control and regulate her anxiety. She uses this type of compulsive defense when she attempts to function adequately.

"She is fearful that her control will break, so she does not permit herself any free emotional participation. She completely represses all her impulses from her consciousness, and in repressing them tries to deny them. She does not even permit herself any phantasy life for fear that her control will break; she now functions as a completely repressed, rigid, emotionally blunted child who fears to react to the environment.

"Dorothy's anxiety stems from her complete unacceptance of herself as a human being. She cannot identify with people, nor accept herself as a person. This unacceptance of herself is related to traumatic experiences with her parental figures. Dorothy views the mother as hard and unyielding, as if made out of stone, unloving, and rejecting. She reacts to the father figure with tremendous anxiety and with extreme fear of authority. She, therefore, excludes this figure from her awareness and is left only with a vague overwhelming fear of all authority as represented by the father figure. Because of her lack of identification with the mother, Dorothy gives some evidence of sexual confusion and conflicts and she is uncertain of the role of her own sex. She does, however, try to relate to people and to the environment, and she is trying to adopt patterns of behavior which will not only make her an acceptable person, but also lessen her anxiety.

"In summary, Dorothy's inability to relate to people, the poor concept of herself, her extreme anxiety, her lack of appropriate affect, and her impaired judgment, are all suggestive of schizophrenia. She is adopting obsessive-compulsive features in order to control the schizophrenic process. She sees herself, as well as the world, as unstable and physically falling apart. She has no emotional cohesiveness. Dorothy's intellectual ability is good, however, and she gives indication of being able to benefit from therapy. Intensive therapy is indicated."

James B.: Age 14, discipline problem

MATHEMATICS TEACHER

"He has improved since the beginning of the term, but his general attitude toward school is poor."

SCIENCE TEACHER

"He has no manners. He is most objectionable to the more fastidious girls because of his constant burping. He tries to tell all he knows at once on a specific subject in spite of the fact that it has no connection with the work. At other times he is silent and doesn't speak at all."

SOCIAL STUDIES TEACHER

"His high IQ does not justify his poor performance. He is a 'weak sister.' "

ENGLISH TEACHER

"He shows a complete lack of respect for both teachers and fellow students. Whenever he has the urge to attend class, it seems to be for the sole purpose of complete disruption of class procedure. He engages students in conversation and attention is completely diverted from the lesson. He seeks the admiration of his peers by being bold, loud, and by using obscene language. While a girl was at the front of the room giving a recitation, he remarked, 'Let me sit closer; I want a better look at her sweater.' A few minutes later he remarked to a neighbor, 'Maybe she wants to f——.' He also asked me sotto voce from his seat, 'Hey, Miss C., do you want to f——?' "

SPANISH TEACHER

"On one of the rare occasions when he decided to attend class he asked for a pass right at the beginning of the period, giving an unsolicited promise that he would return the pass. This should have seemed peculiar to me. However, the prospect of conducting a class without his fatal presence was just too tempting. He has never returned that pass."

PSYCHOLOGICAL REPORT

"James is an impulse-ridden, anxiety-consumed boy who is unable to control his basic aggressive and sexual drives. His lack of judgment and the knowledge that he cannot cope with his impulsiveness results in a basic depression which he tries to repress. His repressive and inhibitory defenses do not operate successfully, however, and James is threatened by conscious depressive feelings.

"The basic conflict appears to center in James's inability to make an adequate sexual identification. He perceives the mother figure as threatening to him. He sees the mother as he sees all females, in an aggressive, foreboding light. Women, to him, are domineering, unloving, ungiving, castrating persons. They belittle the man and in a sense 'rule the world,' as he phrases it. He, too, wants to be domineering and aggressive like women, but he recognizes that he is a male. Men, to him, on the other hand, represent all that is weak and passive in the environment. He sees them as innocuous, undemanding, and assuming secondary roles in society. He therefore denies the male role. Nothing is left for him but to identify with women. He rebels against this identification, however, and so he is torn between two roles and two concepts, neither of which he can accept. Thus he fluctuates between two different roles, attempting in this inadequate way to solve his conflict. The result, however, is only one of depression and extreme feelings of inadequacy. His need for impulsive expression results in behavior which must, of necessity, be completely unacceptable to society. Thus, his acting-out impulses, and the knowledge that they are wrong, only intensifies his feelings of inadequacy, guilt, anxiety, and depression.

"James's intellectual endowment is good. On the Stanford-Binet, Form L, he achieved an IQ of 113, placing him in the bright-normal group of the population. Nevertheless, his emotional conflicts interfere with his intellectual functioning, so that in testing situations, where his achievement is influenced by social judgment, his score is appreciably decreased.

"In summary, James's poor sexual identification, uncontrolled impulsiveness, and poor judgment, result in psychological functioning which must be considered deviate. If immediate therapy is not instituted, the depressive trends so prominent in his personality make-up, coupled with his impulsiveness, may culminate in an agitated depression. Thus, it is possible that he may do violence to himself or to others. He is, therefore, of potential danger to the community."

Judy M.: Age 9, severe discipline problem

ELEMENTARY GRADES TEACHER

"Cries at the slightest provocation. When she doesn't know the lesson, or can't get permission to speak out in class, she has a real tantrum of crying and shouting. Wants to lead all the children, and attempts to do this by bossing them about. When they balk at her efforts, she lashes out at them and engages in a fight. She will even hit the bigger boys in the class. Although she is by no means stupid, she cannot seem to grasp the fundamentals of arithmetic. Her reading, on the other hand, is phenomenally good. Needs constant personal attention from me."

PSYCHOLOGICAL REPORT

"During the testing situation, Judy talked almost constantly in a loud, monotonous tone of voice. She asked questions endlessly: Who took these tests? Why they were taken? How they were scored, etc.?

"Her testing record indicated that despite adequate intelligence (IQ of 93), this girl experiences deep feelings of inadequacy and suffers from overwhelming, disorganizing anxiety. Despite her anxiety, however, she is able to deal with her experiences on a superficial level and maintain some objectivity in her relationship to the environment. Her method of dealing with her anxiety is primarily by putting it at a distance from herself. In attempting to deny her anxiety, she is adopting compulsive mechanisms. This adjustive method, however, is not completely successful, with the result that she reverts to immature, regressive thinking. There is then a marked hiatus between the goals the child sets for herself in her adjustive efforts, and what she achieves. In consequence, she appears to be in a constant state of tension as she strives to maintain whatever stability she can.

"In summary, then, the failure of the compulsive mechanisms to ward off regressive and disorganized reactions point to an extremely infantile level of development. It is possible, although the evidence is not clearly present at this time, that a schizophrenic pathology will develop at some later date."

Robert L.: Age 15, severe discipline problem

ENGLISH TEACHER

"Impossible to handle. Always clowning, very inattentive; everything is a huge joke."

MATHEMATICS TEACHER

"Lazy with little or no interest in his work."

SOCIAL STUDIES TEACHER

"Not passing, does not do assignments. Makes silly faces at the class."

ART TEACHER

"Attitude and work habits very poor. Does not do assignments in class, but delights in drawing dirty pictures and leaving them around so that no one can fail to see them. Looks innocent and hurt when he is accused of drawing them."

SCIENCE TEACHER

"Destroys equipment with the greatest of ease. Other children, particularly girls, complain about his behavior. They say he pinches them although I never caught him at it."

PSYCHOLOGICAL REPORT

"Robert came to the testing situation with a sneer on his lips and a superficial bravado he really did not feel. His latent anxiety became more in evidence as the testing progressed, with the result that at the conclusion of the session he was verbally assaultive to the examiner.

"On the Wechsler-Bellevue Intelligence Scale, Form I, Robert achieved an IQ of 106, indicating that he is functioning at an average intellectual level.

"On the projective material, Robert gave a picture of a severe homosexual conflict which is at present at an unconscious level, but which threatens to come into consciousness. In his desperate attempts to deny this conflict, he distorts reality and conjures up a phantasy with which he can cope. He then fluctuates between a reality which he shares with others and a phantasy world of his own.

"His conflict concerning homosexuality is centered about his difficulty at maintaining the male role. He wants very much to play the passive role, but because he fears his passivity and his homosexuality, he overcompensates by overaggressive behavior. This behavior is most often directed toward women whom he views with extreme hatred. He cannot admit his overaggression, however, so he projects it onto others, believing that others hate him, and, indeed, persecute him. Thus, paranoid elements are present.

"Because of this boy's distortions of reality, his poor sexual identification, and his paranoid thinking, the diagnosis of schizophrenia must be made."

Dolores S.: Age 10, no discipline problem,
considered well adjusted by the teacher

ELEMENTARY GRADES TEACHER

"She is satisfactory, a very slow learner, but in a group in which many pupils are slow, she is adequate. Never causes any trouble. A well-behaved child. Seems to be well adjusted because she is so quiet."

PSYCHOLOGICAL REPORT

"This child was eager to co-operate during the testing session. Her manner was pleasant, compliant, and co-operative. When, however, she failed on test items, she evidenced marked anxiety. This was most prominent in situations involving concrete manipulative materials.

"The results of the psychological tests indicate a very limited, barren personality structure. This girl has no way of dealing with her experiences except in a stereotyped fashion. There is no capacity for enriching her experiences and setting up mutually satisfying interpersonal relationships. Similarly, there is only a slight capacity for phantasy.

"She is aware, however, of her limitations and of the emotional aspects of the environment. She would like to do something about it, but is unable to achieve this except on a most infantile level. In the face of emotionally charged situations, she becomes disorganized in a way that strongly suggests that she is suffering from an organic disorder.

"This organic disorder is again clearly indicated by her handling of manipulative materials. She scored a verbal IQ of 109, and a performance IQ of 85. Although her full scale IQ is obviously average or better (97), the disparity between the verbal IQ and the performance IQ indicates an organic difficulty. In addition, there were many evidences of poor visual perception and deficient visual-motor responses, all of which were suggestive of an organic malfunctioning.

"The child tries to compensate for her inadequacy by adapting a conforming, pleasant manner. But this façade proves too much for her at times, and she is forced to admit her difficulties and inadequacies. At these times, her anxiety reaches an agitated state.

"Diagnosis: Organic malfunctioning. Recommendation: A physical and neurological examination.

("This child was later given a complete physical work-up and was found to have been suffering from lesions of the brain.")

Too often, teachers misunderstand the behavior of children in their classes. Children who are particularly aggressive may be considered merely "bad," "fresh," or "lazy," rather than disturbed, while children who are unusually quiet are often thought to be well behaved and well adjusted. The importance of being aware of the shy, quiet child who does not participate in classroom activities, who finds it difficult to respond to questions, and who has few friends, should not be minimized. On the other hand, the teacher, often painfully aware of the aggressive, demanding child, should also understand that extreme aggression may be symptomatic of maladjustment.

SUMMARY

While the detection of maladjustment in children is the responsibility of all adults, the teacher is in the most favored position of all to note any abnormality of behavior. It is the teacher who spends the greatest amount of time with the child, and it is the teacher who can observe the child not only as an individual, but also in relation to the school group. Thus the teacher must bear a large part of the responsibility for noting evidences of emotional disturbance as manifested in behavior, and for recommending further psychological study. If such observations and referrals were made a regular part of the school program, perhaps many of the disturbed youngsters who later find their way to children's courts because of their bizarre and hostile behavior, could be helped before any tragedy occurs. The educational system, in this sense, can and should act as a preventive force.

Chapter II

The Schizophrenic Child

The most deviate form of emotional disturbance is labeled *psychosis*. In general terms, it may be stated that a psychosis is in evidence when reality is so painful to an individual that he escapes from it and substitutes a new reality to take its place. The remodeled reality is then accepted as actual fact, and behavior is patterned in relationship to this new reality, which exists only for the individual concerned. In psychosis then, an individual creates new perceptions to conform to this new reality, which in turn may give rise to symptoms such as bizarre behavior, delusional systems, hallucinations, exaggeratedly egocentric thinking, and falsifications of memory. Thus, if a person suffers from delusions, he may believe himself to be the reincarnation of some historic person. If he suffers from either visual or auditory hallucinations, he may see things which no one else can see, or he may hear sounds or voices which no one else hears. Both hallucinations and delusions are distortions of reality. Moreover, they are indications of bizarre, distorted thinking processes which are peculiar to the individual and reflective of his own emotional problems. It is indeed difficult to characterize psychosis by an exact formula, but on a descriptive level it is possible to say that in all cases of schizophrenia the following elements are present: "strangeness and bizarre nature of the symptoms, absurdity and unpredictability of the affects and intellectual ideas, and the obviously inadequate connection between these two." [1] Thus, to give an

---

[1] O. Fenichel, *The Psychoanalytic Theory of Neurosis* (New York: W. W. Norton and Co., 1945), p. 415.

example, a patient may experience feelings of persecution (bizarreness of symptom), but he may speak about these feelings with a smile on his face or with an apparent unconcern (inadequate and inappropriate connection between the idea and the feeling expressed).

SCHIZOPHRENIA IN CHILDHOOD

The literature related to the psychoses of childhood is characterized by varying views regarding the etiological basis of the schizophrenic process. The major differences appear to center on whether this illness is constitutional and stems from an inherent biological defect, or whether it is functional and therefore psychogenic in nature. Is the psychotic child one of normal potential, emotionally distorted by psychic traumas, or does this child start life with defective potential which makes for a constitution incapable of adjustment?

Although research from either point of view has acknowledged evidence supporting the other, the old "nature vs. nurture" dichotomy forms the essential difference between the two concepts. Investigators like Lauretta Bender, a pioneer and one of the foremost authorities in the field, believe that schizophrenia is a biological phenomenon determined before birth, probably by hereditary factors, and activated by some physiological crisis like puberty, severe illness, or birth itself.[2] According to Bender, schizophrenia is a clinical entity which manifests pathology in all areas of behavior which function through the central nervous system. These areas include the automatic control of the body, motor behavior, perceptual patterning, intellectual functioning, and emotional maturation.[3] Bender suggests that the biologic defect known as schizophrenia stems from the inability of the child to discard the primitive motility of the embryonic state.[4] According to this view, the primary and specific symptomatology of childhood schizophrenia is derived from the plasticity of the embryo. The growing child is seen as unable to construct mature patterns of behavior because he is incapable of discarding the primitive motility pattern with which he

---

[2] L. Bender, "Childhood Schizophrenia," *Psychiatric Quarterly*, XVII (1953), p. 68.
[3] *Loc. cit.*
[4] L. Bender, "The Schizophrenic Child," in H. Michael-Smith, *Pediatric Problems in Clinical Practice* (New York: Grune and Stratton, 1954), p. 52.

started uterine life. Although the schizophrenic child cannot make
progressively mature adaptations, he nevertheless frequently shows a
precocity or a talent for an adaptational process far beyond his years
and on a high artistic level. This phenomenon is explained as an over-
compensatory mechanism for his biologic defect. It is also a defense
against the disintegrating force of the pathology itself. According to
Bender, therefore, precocity or spurts of development found in schizophrenic children are merely evidences of uneven growth patterns.[5]
Thus, some children are regressive, retarded, inhibited, autistic, withdrawn, psychically underdeveloped, and overly concrete in their thinking. These children are demonstrating "developmental lags" in their
maturation process. On the other hand, there are children who are
precocious, overactive, overdeveloped, highly articulate, overrelated to
others, and excessively abstract in their thinking. These children show
the spurts of development. While some schizophrenic children go
through phases of both extremes of behavior, most show a mixture of
these extremes. Schizophrenic children, therefore, may appear to be
retarded in some areas and overdeveloped or precocious in others.

Bender describes the schizophrenic child as a creature of extremes,
not only in behavior, but in physical appearance.[6] Physically, he is too
small for his age or too big; too fat or too thin; or too flaccid or too
rigid in muscle tone. Similarly, in behavior he is too aggressive or too
withdrawn, too active or too apathetic. This child is so threatened by
these reactive mechanisms which are beyond his control that he responds in a manner characteristic of schizophrenic children: he suffers
from intense anxiety. The disorganization arising from the schizophrenic process itself interferes with the functioning of the personality
and the development of the ego.

The schizophrenic personality, therefore, has difficulty in establishing and maintaining an ego. Adherents of the biologic school attribute
this lack of ego functioning to biological, and possibly even hereditary
factors. On the other hand, the psychoanalytic schools attribute the

---

[5] L. Bender, "Childhood Schizophrenia," *American Journal of Orthopsychiatry*, XVII
(1947), 40–56.
[6] *Loc. cit.*

lack of ego functioning primarily to environmental or psychogenic factors. There is no rigid dichotomy between the two schools, however,
and adherents of both schools frequently agree that psychogenic and
biologic factors are both important etiological considerations.

Schizophrenia, considered from a purely psychoanalytic point of view,
rests primarily—as does all analytic theory—on the hypotheses that
were originally developed by Freud. His psychology was one of motivation and dealt primarily with the unconscious. According to Freud,
the child at birth and in infancy cannot distinguish between the identity
of his personal self and the configuration that is the environment.[7] As
the child develops he explores his own identity and begins to know and
experience the self as discrete from the environment. People in the
environment and objects of the environment start to assume their own
reality. This conscious self, in Freud's terminology, is called the ego.
In addition to the ego, Freud defined the id and the superego as parts
of the personality. The id, he hypothesized, is the unconscious which
contains the drives, instincts, and urges common to all individuals and
which must be controlled. The superego is the controller—that part of
a person which is commonly referred to as the conscience.

Ego development begins at birth. It proceeds from the stage of complete fetal dependence to some form of independence. As an infant, the
baby is all powerful, having all his needs gratified immediately by his
mother. His dependence is, therefore, an expression of both power and
weakness. As he matures, however, he relinquishes some of the power,
becomes a more independently functioning organism, and has less
need for others to supply his gratification. In this process of going
from dependency to independence, of relinquishing omnipotence for
socialization, his ego develops—that is, he becomes aware of himself
as an individual.

The very young child is unable to differentiate between his own
body boundaries and the world about him. He cannot differentiate
between the me-ness of himself and environment. He does not know
where his body ends and the environment begins. In this undifferen-

---

[7] Fenichel, *op. cit.*, p. 35.

tiated state of body awareness, the infant feels at one with the mother's body, treating it as if it were his own body. As the child matures, he develops an ability to separate his own body from his mother's and to differentiate between himself and his environment. He develops a perceptive awareness of the environment. This stage in ego development is a very vulnerable one, as it is the beginning awareness of reality.

In analytic terms, childhood schizophrenia is seen as a problem in ego development, originating in infancy and predisposing individuals to remain alienated from reality. From this frame of reference, two clinically distinct categories of childhood schizophrenia may be differentiated: autistic and symbiotic.

Autistic schizophrenia is characterized by unawareness. The mother, as representative of the outside world, never seems to have been perceived emotionally as a separate entity. The child is unaware of the mother just as he is unaware of the environment. Consequently, he is unable to identify himself as an individual and, as a result, he is incapable of making adequate interpersonal relationships.

In the symbiotic type of schizophrenia, the mother-infant relationship is so marked, that the mother does not become separated from the self. The mother's body is perceived to be in unity with the child's body. The child clings to the mother with a strong physical attachment, almost melting into the mother's body. This melting is described by Bender as a lag in the developmental curve, wherein the child is still reacting as an infant instead of on a level commensurate with his physical and maturational age.[8] The world is hostile and threatening to the child and anxiety concerning separation from his mother overwhelms him. His anxiety reactions are intense and diffuse. There are severe panic reactions at the thought of separation. He too, therefore, is incapable of identifying himself as an adequate human being and consequently cannot relate adequately to others.

Behaviorally there are subtle differences between the two types of schizophrenia. The autistic schizophrenic child is unyielding. He does

---

[8] L. Bender, *loc. cit.*

not seek close physical contact. In fact, he avoids any contact, because he does not perceive people as distinct from the environment. He, himself, has no awareness of himself as a human being, and, therefore, has no concept of other human beings. On the other hand, the symbiotic schizophrenic child seeks all human contact. Because he is so uncertain of his own ego identification, he searches for it in relationship to others. He develops a close, physical clinging relationship to the mother or a mother substitute. In his attempts to be a part of the other person's body, he tries to find an identity and ego of his own. Thus, the symbiotic child is often imitative in speech, manner, or even thought, attempting in this way to find the identity he could not establish within himself.

BEHAVIOR PATTERNS OF THE SCHIZOPHRENIC CHILD

The following examples are behavioral descriptions of schizophrenic children who were hospitalized for observation and who attended school in a psychiatric hospital during their observation period.[9] No attempt is made to discuss the dynamic mechanisms and causative factors, nor is there a necessity to relate each case to theoretical formulations of the various schools of psychiatry. Rather, the following cases are descriptive of the manifest behavior of the schizophrenic child who is obviously psychotic and disoriented and easily recognized as grossly deviate. These children represent the severest form of psychosis, living in a world of their own, losing contact with reality as others perceive it, and behaving in a bizarre, distorted matter.

Margaret D.: Female, Age 9, Normal IQ

Throughout her stay at the psychiatric hospital, Margaret made no attempts at verbal contact, either with adults or children. She did not respond when spoken to and completely ignored her environment except to strike out brutally at others without provocation. She was hyperactive, moving around the room constantly without ever sitting still. She was incontinent, and gave no evidence of any of the usual needs like hunger or

---

[9] Most of the children discussed in this chapter were patients in Bellevue Psychiatric Hospital and attended, while in the hospital, a New York City Board of Education School, which is part of the "600" Schools Division designed particularly for emotionally disturbed children. The school is situated in the hospital building.

thirst. She hallucinated openly, talking to herself and spitting out at anything, anybody, or nothing. She was completely destructive, throwing, breaking, or tearing any objects she managed to get hold of, as well as consistently tearing her own clothing from her body. She would not permit anyone to come near her or touch her. Most of her physical needs, therefore, such as washing or hair combing, were neglected. The only acceptable activity in which she ever engaged, although sporadically and unevenly was drawing and painting. At these times, she was able to respond to verbal questions with a monosyllabic reply. Her paintings seemed to be her only contact with reality, and through them she occasionally made contact for a moment with the environment. The art work she produced represented the distorted perceptions she experienced and the disorganizing process which was present in all her functioning. Her figures were bizarre, floating in space, and indicative of her own feelings of disorientation. The entire impression was one of complete disorganization.

Robert S.: Male, Age 14, IQ 102

Robert was incapable of making any adequate interpersonal relationships. He could not participate in any form of social intercourse, not even simple conversation. If left alone, he would sit and stare into space for hours. His movements were erratic, impulsive, and inappropriate in that after sitting for hours rigidly, he would suddenly gesticulate, making grimaces, or dart from the classroom without provocation. He was extremely passive in relationship to adult figures, following commands to the point of unreality. For example, when he was told to sit and read a book, he would stare at the book until he was specifically told to stop. It could not be determined whether or not he could actually read. Distracting events about him, the ringing of bells, or the shouting of children, did not affect his apparent concentration on the task before him. He would stop only when the same adult who set the task initially before him insisted that he stop. He had no relationship with his peers other than inarticulate grunting when provoked by them. Occasionally, this grunting would be accompanied by a methodical removal of all his clothing. The only indication he gave of recognizing the identity of another individual was his need to remain physically close to them. He frequently spoke to himself and seemed to be carrying on a conversation with an imaginary person.

Marie B.: Female, Age 7

Marie was a completely disoriented, confused child, who made no contact with anyone. She gesticulated wildly with her arms and her eyes darted constantly without any real perception of the environment. She seemed frightened, cried almost continuously and appeared very anxious. Marie seemed to be hallucinating, responding to inner stimuli and evidencing fear of imaginary things. She never spoke to another child nor played with any of the toys in the room. When handed a plaything, she became panic-stricken and engaged in violent destruction. She could not care for her bodily needs, soiling and wetting herself without being aware of it.

It is obvious from these three behavioral descriptions of psychotic children that they were not able to contact reality as it is perceived by most children. They were, therefore, living in a world of their own creation. These children would have been considered very disturbed and labeled psychotic, insane, or abnormal, by even the most psychologically unoriented.

Pre-Psychosis Personality Patterns

While psychotic behavior which is constantly unrealistic and bizarre over a long period of time is easily diagnosed, there are those children whose bizarreness appears suddenly and/or episodically. These are the children who are able to maintain contact with reality until such time as their superficial hold upon this reality breaks and they become psychotic. These children are disturbed and have tendencies toward psychotic breakdowns even while they manage to behave in a way that most people would consider within the normal range. A trained observer, however, would have recognized behavioral deviations, such as unrealistic anxiety, depression, withdrawal, or overcompliance, which had been manifested by these children even while they appeared to be "normal." Before a child becomes overtly psychotic, there is usually some evidence of malfunctioning or maladjustment. The following cases illustrate the apparent sudden onset of the psychosis, and the underlying maladjustments which preceded it.

Helen D.: Female, Age 11, IQ 98

This girl made good superficial relationships with both children and adults. She participated in classroom activities and was interested in academic work. Her record from the regular school in the community indicated that Helen had fairly good academic achievement, adequate social relationships, and seemed to be functioning adequately. Her absence record was high, however, and indicated that she seemed susceptible to many illnesses. Her mother stated that Helen was a delicate child who complained of physical illnesses, for which, frequently, there seemed to be no apparent cause. At home she was considered well adjusted, quiet, obedient, shy, serious, and well trained, a child who seemed to enjoy staying at home and who appeared to be devoted to her parents. Suddenly, without apparent cause, Helen began to refuse to walk alone in the street. She became fearful of attack by imaginary wild animals and she was terrified that the streets would open up and permit the devil to attack her. She refused to enter the school playground, openly expressing her fear of animals, death, open streets and poisoned food. She soon began to believe she was being poisoned. In the hospital school, her behavior seemed to be that of a "normal" child except for the fact that she refused all refreshments, verbalizing her fear that she was being poisoned by the teacher, and at those times she would hallucinate openly.

Mary M.: Female, Age 14, IQ 99

Mary was a model student in school. She received good grades and superior ratings in deportment. She was described as co-operative, quiet, shy, and easy to get along with. She had no friends, but this was attributed to the fact that her interest was in schoolwork and keeping house for her mother, who worked to support a fatherless home. She was a passive, compliant, well-liked child, who was rarely gay, spoke only when spoken to, smiled, but never laughed, and who was never obtrusive. Mary always prepared her schoolwork and conformed to all school rules. Suddenly, without any apparent external reason, she stopped doing her schoolwork and became so withdrawn and depressed that it was evident she was not really aware of her surroundings a good bit of the time. She became preoccupied; her attention wandered, and her concern centered about her own private thoughts. She was preoccupied with a fear of death, not only for herself, but for her mother. Her anxiety became so intolerable and overwhelming that she attempted suicide.

In the two cases presented the actual onset of the psychosis was very sudden. When the case histories and personality development patterns of these two girls were carefully examined, however, it became clear that they had a history of extreme passivity, overcompliance, and depression. Psychosis which seemed to appear suddenly was actually preceded by a history of maladjustment, the symptoms of which went unrecognized. The withdrawal patterns of these two girls characterize the shy, compliant child who may be just as disturbed as the most aggressive child.

There are, however, children who are similarly disturbed, but who may not be consistently withdrawn. Overtly, they react quite normally to the classroom situation until a moment comes when they engage in bizarre, erratic behavior in a very sporadic, ephemeral way. Such children are able to function satisfactorily, getting along well with children, making fairly adequate relations with the teacher, and maintaining normal academic standards. Their behavior seems normal until they suddenly defy the set pattern of the school structure by what seems to be a temporary infraction of school regulations. At such times they may seem to be very silly, act without rhyme or reason, and have momentary high nuisance value. This behavior might consist of such acts as suddenly climbing on top of the wardrobe without reason, darting from the room without apparent reason, hiding behind a piece of furniture, leaping from desk to desk, pretending to be an animal, etc.

This type of behavior is obviously bizarre, but because such behavior is infrequent and ephemeral, it is quickly forgotten until it recurs. When bizarre behavior is not in evidence, the child is apparently conforming within normal, accepted limits. This type of behavior should be taken seriously and calls for psychological investigation.

The following two cases are examples of momentary behavioral bizarreness.

Ralph Q.: Male, Age 9, IQ 105

Ralph Q. was a happy, pleasant-looking boy who was compliant and quiet in the classroom. He was not a good student and was failing in reading, but he accepted his difficulty and worked hard at overcoming his deficiency. He had some close friends and gave a superficial picture of a normal, average child. Occasionally, however, he would, without permission and without any evidence of provocation, dart from the room and immediately disappear into the hall. When others were sent to look for him, he would be found on another floor, idly wandering about the school building. He would return to the classroom willingly, could not remember having left the room, and could offer no explanation for his behavior.

Raoul M.: Male, Age 11, IQ 99

Raoul was a solemn, serious child who was somewhat retarded academically, but who seemed otherwise able to conform to expected patterns of behavior. Every once in a while he would suddenly climb on the window sill and leap from there to a desk some distance away. When asked why he did this he would laugh and say he was an airplane. He resumed his usual normalcy almost immediately, not at all concerned about the ridicule the other children heaped upon him.

These two illustrations were taken from school records of children who, when their bizarreness increased, were placed in a psychiatric hospital where they were diagnosed as schizophrenic. Fleeting bizarre behavior is often ignored in school until such time as the behavior becomes completely unrealistic.

BIZARRE IDEATION AND VERBALIZATIONS

Bizarre behavior may appear in conjunction with a special type of verbalization which, although sporadic, is nevertheless an additional indication of maladjustment. These verbalizations are the overt manifestations of psychotic thinking processes, and indicate, in some small measure, the confusion and distortion of reality which the child is inwardly experiencing. During the course of a normal conversation, for example, a child's distorted thinking can so intrude upon the reality of the situation that the verbalizations become a confused mixture of reality and irrationality.

Tony C.: Male, Age 15, IQ 107

Tony was academically retarded, giving the impression of defective functioning in spite of a high normal IQ. He was admitted to the hospital by the recommendation of the court where he was sent for truancy. His school record indicated that prior to the onset of truancy he presented no particular problems, was liked by both teachers and children, and was getting along in a homogeneous group of dull children. In the hospital school he showed compliant obedience, co-operated fully with directions, and manifested no overt psychotic behavior. His thinking processes, however, did give indication of confusion of thought, flight of ideas, and contamination of reality. The following composition was written after a group discussion about the meaning of Armistice Day:

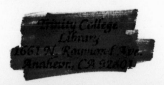

"It better be peace for a while because another war would be real bad as the comic books make out, not so fantastic, but real bad. There will be atom bombs dropped on everybody. Nothing will stop it. We got lots of defense and even balloons on the West Coast won't be enough. We got atomic cannons and guns and we got some we don't even know about that we are saving for the Third World War. It will be pretty messy. We won't be sending any help to any country because we'll be needing it ourselves. I thought that just like when Columbus discovered America that was a dangerous journey, but now when you travel back and forth it's a pleasure. Maybe it sounds fantastic now but a vacation on Mars would be accomplished before I get so old. Or going to the North Pole or some South Sea Island would be all right, but I guess that's no good 'cause they'll bomb everywhere if it's a real war. Maybe by the time the Third World War comes, 25 years from now, there will be space travel and we could get to the moon or Mars or Venus. That's the day I'm waiting for, I'll open a travel agency and have a sign in the window, "Pleasure Cruises to Mars."

It is apparent from this story that this boy's thought processes centered upon a reality situation which he could not maintain. The insinuations of his phantasy were so pervasive that, even with a basic realistic thread of an idea, he took off into a bizarre flight of ideas. The flight of ideas is very apparent in the thought processes of disturbed children, and frequently is one of the symptoms of schizophrenia. The child may start with a rational, logical thought, but because he becomes so stimulated by all the associations that each thought or word produces, he fluctuates from idea to idea in rapid association, losing the logic of the original idea. The following extract, including a composition written by a schizophrenic boy, age nine, demonstrates clearly how one idea stimulates another, resulting in an illogical sequence of ideas.

Edward M.: Male, Age 9, IQ 103

Edward came to the hospital with his brother after their parents had been charged with neglect for permitting the children to wander indiscriminately in the neighborhood at all hours of the day and night. Edward was considered a discipline problem in school, truanting and exhibiting aggressive behavior. He was not described by any school record as a possible maladjusted child, although, in addition to truancy and aggressiveness,

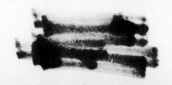

he was a non-reader. His thought processes were quite unusual in that he tended to confuse animate and inanimate things. He was preoccupied with macabre phantasy, with stories of Frankenstein, Dracula, the devil, bloodsuckers, witches, and bats. He liked to paint and would only paint morbid subjects even when asked to paint something else. His paintings were overpoweringly aggressive.

Even in academic areas he could not be diverted from his preoccupations with phantasy figures. He refused to learn to read until reading was approached through the utilization of bizarre material. His reading consisted of stories of Frankenstein, Dracula, etc., which he invented. He made very good superficial contact with both adults and children and was described as delightful and charming by authority figures. If the relationship continued, however, it was evident that it had no real meaning to him. There was no real understanding of the intrinsic value of any real emotional affect. He always seemed completely happy, meeting both praise and criticism with an unrealistic euphoria. The following story was dictated by him in response to a request to tell about an incident in his childhood.

"When I was little, yes, when I was little, I was a boy. One day I was waiting for my mother to come home because she used to work and I used to wait. And so I got mad when she didn't come home. So I thought she'll be sorry and she wouldn't find me because I used to like to play in the refrigerator with my little brother. Only he wasn't there and he was with my grandmother. So I poured myself into the ice cube box but first I made myself into water and then went into the freezer. She was mad because she couldn't find me because all the time I was ice, so she looked but she got thirsty and she went to the icebox and poured me down the drain."

Upon completion of the story, Edward looked up a bit startled, laughed, and walked over to a table and started to draw.

Edward's thought processes, his concern with the supernatural, and his macabre art productions are all obviously bizarre. His self-concept is so obviously weak and his confusion of animate and inanimate objects so bizarre, that they indicate a gross distortion of realistic thinking.

Patricia K.: Female, Age 11, IQ 95

Patricia was a child who functioned well in academic areas and presented no distortion of overt behavior. Her rich phantasy life was in evidence only when her thought processes and imaginative capacities were permitted free rein. The following is a composition she wrote in response to the title "My Ambition."

"I wish I could live in candy land so I could have all the cotton candy, lollypops, ice cream sodas and strawberry short cake. I would also like to go to pencil land.

"Once I lived in pencil land and I was a pencil too. When I was a pencil I was owned by a little boy. He bit me and I just had to scream. I told him about pencil land. Then he said to me, 'Would you take me to pencil land?' So I took him. He saw pencils marching. They were in prison. The pencil sharpener came running after them. The little boy dropped a piece of iron on the sharpener. It broke. The pencils said, 'Thank you for saving our lives.'"

Not only does this production indicate bizarre phantasy, but also a confabulatory flight of ideas.

Walter T.: Male, Age 9, IQ 86

In the regular grades, Walter was a hyperactive, restless child who seemed to need excessive attention. He could not read or write and had no arithmetic concepts. He made good relationships in the school and had many friends. He seemed to be a happy child who could interest himself in many academic activities even though he met with no success. The teacher considered him a dull child who needed special attention.

During his stay at the hospital school he gave no indication of problem behavior. He participated freely in all activities and began to learn to read. Suddenly one day in the midst of a painting session he asked for materials to make a box. After he made and painted the box, which he constructed to look like a phonograph, he announced that he was a radio. He began to announce the news. The following is a verbatim record of his news broadcast:

"Here's two hundred men missing from a warehouse. There was a robbery last night. Superman came. There was two hundred missing. The record player man says send two hundred movies to the record player to-night. So many people got killed in Washington to Brooklyn. When they got killed they sent two hundred Army men. They sent two hundred girls over to Washington. The cops said they would send two hundred men. Two hundred thousand dollars was missing last night. They got two hundred Cadillacs. They got hot dogs and new houses. Everyone is glad they got new houses."

Both of the above productions show a bizarre flight of ideas. Patricia started with a realistic topic but ended with a complete change of thought. Similarly, Walter's verbal productions are so unstable that they leap from one thought to another without logical sequence. Walter also perseverated to the number two hundred, using it indiscriminately and without real meaning. Both examples indicate a confusion of thought of which these children were completely unaware.

Distortions are found not only in ideas but in the formulation of isolated words and phrases. Disturbed children frequently like to play with the sounds of letters and words, making up alliterative and rhyming words and phrases which have no connection with each other in thought. The sheer sounds delight the children, and stimulate them to continue their productions and elaborate upon them. For example, the following word play was recorded at a time when Robert, age ten, was involved in decorating the classroom for Christmas. He kept up a chant as he painted a Christmas mural. The following excerpt illustrates this play upon words:

"Christmas, Christ, Wistmas, Wiste, misy, misy tree. Popcorn string, popcorn bing, wing, witch, rich, bitch, popcorn bitch, popcorn bitch, popcorn pitch, popcorn bitch. Teacher is a popcorn bitch, teacher is a popcorn bitch."

Similarly, another child's productions were recorded as follows. They are a play upon a name.

"Isabel, Jezebel, went to her friendzabel. Friendzabel, Isabel had a big Jezebel. Jezebel, friendzabel, Isabel, wizabel, madabel, tedabel, Jezebel, Isabel."

The need to emphasize this type of production is particularly necessary because frequently such word play may indicate serious disturbance even though no other obvious overt behavior symptoms are discernible. Schilder believes that word play indicates a regression to a period of primitive aggressiveness.[10] Such word play should be investigated if it persists, particularly if the child cannot be made aware that he is being silly or talking nonsense. The following conversation is a

---

[10] Paul Schilder, *Goals and Desires of Man* (New York: Columbia University Press, 1942), p. 37.

verbatim report of three children who engaged in word play which not only had serious significance to them, but, also, through which they seemed to be communicating with each other in a kind of special language:

John, age 9, Seon, age 9, and Irene, age 11, were drawing when a teacher, Mr. Kaufman, was mentioned aloud by another child.

JOHN: Mr. Kaufman has kauf in his pants.

SEON: Kauf, kauf, pauf, pauf.

JOHN: You have kauf in your pants, Irene.

IRENE: Give me a bauf.

JOHN: No, I'll give you a belch.

SEON: Shut up, you belch after you eat frankfurters.

IRENE: Shut up you two frankfurters. Now we present the two Belgian frankfurters!

The significance of such conversation is apparent not only in the experimentation with sounds, but, also, in the seemingly real communication of ideas in a series of nonsense words which are grammatically so constructed that the total picture appears to be adequate, meaningful language. There are appropriate inflections, pauses for thought, and the whole conversation takes on the characteristics of acceptable social intercourse. However, the fact remains that the conversation is actually meaningless, the words are incomprehensible, and the entire situation is bizarre.

Another form of word play is the actual application of new meaning to old words or putting words in combination with each other, thereby distorting the meaning of the whole. The words have specific meaning to the individual child and are an expression of a concept which he has originated. For instance, a disturbed boy described another child who was openly masturbating as "playing with his magic stern." When asked what the word *stern* meant, he replied, "You know," and he drew a picture of a penis. Although both *magic* and *stern* are perfectly acceptable, ordinary words, when used in this context they represent thinking which is unique to this child because they are imbued with a meaning of which only he is aware.

Another example is the child who was describing adults by giving them rather distinctive labels. He called a person he liked "a witch"; the next preference in his affection was called "a frog"; and the one he disliked at the moment was called "nothing but a box of Swans-down Cake Flour." When called upon to explain, he said that a witch was good because it was almost human, and even better than human because it could fly; a frog was all right because it was alive, even if not human, and a frog could jump; but a box of cake flour was just "plain dead."

Verbal play is common to many young children with fairly good intellectual endowment, and can be both charming and imaginative. However, when this highly imaginative process becomes constant and bizarre, and is invested with a kind of peculiar personal meaning, it must be considered a mechanism of unrealistic psychotic behavior.

SUMMARY

Psychosis is characterized by a break with reality. Words take on special personal meaning, and reality has little value in comparison to inner thoughts. The islands of reality to which the psychotic child sometimes seems to have access may be disarming to the observer and may obscure psychological malfunctioning. The observer, however, must be on the alert to detect behavior which is symptomatic of malad-justment, even though that behavior is seemingly insignificant.

Chapter III

Detecting Symptoms of Organic
Malfunctioning in Children

For the purposes of this chapter, diffuse organic malfunctioning refers to brain or central nervous system trauma without any gross neurological damage, in which case a diagnosis of organic malfunctioning can be deduced only by extensive examination and behavioral observations. This definition excludes from consideration injuries which have specific sequelae, such as brain malformation with concomitant gross motor disturbances, developmental defects of brain substance as are associated with endogenous mental deficiency, or any brain injury which fits a particular clinical syndrome such as Little's disease or Sydenham's chorea. Diagnosing for minimal organic malfunctioning can be a most difficult task because there may be no clearly defined evidence of neurological damage, or because the evidence is very slight and inconclusive.

Frequently, children with minimal injury show no specific signs of neurological malfunction or damage. Occasionally, they may show evidences of some very minor signs which in themselves do not fall into any disease entity. In fact, symptoms of neurological malfunctioning, to be significant, must be related to chronological age before they can be considered meaningful. In addition, they must be supported by tests of all kinds before organic malfunctioning can be determined.

BEHAVIORAL DEVIATIONS OF THE CHILD WITH BRAIN INJURY

The need for diagnosing diffuse organic malfunctioning in children who do not show any particular obvious neurological symptomatology is brought about, almost always, by overt unacceptable behavior which society refuses to tolerate. This behavior, although resembling other forms of behavior maladjustment, is primarily the result of some organic damage rather than psychogenic or neurotic factors.

Organic malfunctioning can give rise to behavior which is erratic, un-co-ordinated, uncontrolled, uninhibited, and socially unacceptable. There may be hyperactivity and disinhibition, periods of extreme elation, explosive crying, and helplessness and despair in the face of a problem which is not beyond the child's level of knowledge or ability. There are evidences of malfunctioning in tasks involving visual motor co-ordination. Children who are organically damaged frequently cannot copy accurately geometric designs such as squares, diamonds, or triangles. They have difficulty drawing straight lines, crosses, and angular figures. They are notably poor in arts and crafts, and unco-ordinated in athletics. Behaviorally, organically damaged children frequently perseverate a response. For instance, they may be unable to stop laughing even when all reason for it is removed, or they may move a toy about in an automatic manner for as long as an hour at a time.

The child who is suffering from some diffuse organic disturbance is differentiated with great difficulty from the schizophrenic child, the neurotic child, or the psychopath. He may resemble the neurotic child in that he may display excessive anxiety, or there may be an emotional shallowness present that resembles the "not caring" of the full-blown psychopath. The child who is organically damaged can also display the "flight of ideas" and irrelevant thinking of the schizophrenic child, and may seem to be incapable of making adequate interpersonal relationships. It takes a really sensitive and experienced diagnostician to recognize the subtle qualitative shades of differences between these groups, and differential diagnosis cannot be made without the information provided by psychological tests, particularly those tests requiring motor co-ordination.

PERCEPTUAL AND CONCEPTUAL DEVIATIONS

When subjected to tests, the sensory motor performance of the child with organic malfunctioning indicates a lack of integration in the perceptual field as compared to an organically normal group, and it is through this area of functioning that a differential diagnosis can frequently be made. The tests of the organically damaged child show a distortion of patterns, a confusion of background with configurations in the foreground, and an inability to perceive forms both tactually and visually. In addition, testing may indicate that perseveration is prevalent, particularly when visual patterns are presented for reproduction that involve motor performance.

Tests for conceptual relationships indicate that organically damaged children are unable to abstract and organize, and that they tend toward stereotyped perseverative responses. They give evidences of incoherence, confabulation, and emphasis upon unessential details. The disorders of thinking and reasoning in the child with a diffuse organic disturbance seem to be very similar to the thinking disorders of the schizophrenic child. Their concept formations may be bizarre, and their aberrant thought processes tend toward overlooking rather obvious relationships and explaining the oversight with fantastic rationalizations. The organically damaged child may try to compensate for his disabilities by rushing into experiences in an ill-considered, impulsive fashion, resulting in inappropriate reactions; or he may, instead, constantly protest his inability to deal with a situation, and request an inordinate amount of help and reassurance. Here, again, a differentiation between the schizophrenic process and organic malfunctioning is often difficult to make. The child with an organic disturbance, however, is usually not negativistic, and generally attempts to fulfill the task before him. The organically damaged child, moreover, frequently expresses his feelings of complete and utter helplessness, and seeks constant support.

DETECTING ORGANIC MALFUNCTIONING IN THE CLASSROOM

Learning for the organically damaged child is a more difficult problem than for most children with equivalent intellectual endowment. In addition to the usual problems of learning which all children face, the organically damaged child must somehow compensate for his impediment. The uninhibited impulsiveness of the organically damaged child is the result of many undifferentiated, uncontrollable drives which the child experiences. This child makes many uncontrolled random movements; he cannot concentrate; he is hypersensitive to stimuli in the environment; he has distorted perceptions; and he sometimes manifests poorly integrated thinking. These many factors add to the learning problem.

Children who suffer from diffuse organic malfunctioning overrespond to stimuli in the environment. The child who is attempting to read may be distracted by a picture in a book and become so concerned with a minor detail of the drawing, or the color, that the reading activity is lost.

Reading is not an isolated problem, but rather a further manifestation of perceptual difficulties confronting organically damaged children. Poor visual perceptions give rise to reversals in letters, words, and phonograms. There is poor differentiation in speech sounds. The child, therefore, may have extreme difficulty in learning how to read if the teaching approach is only through visual methods.

Cursive writing is perhaps the most outstandingly difficult task for organically damaged children to learn. The fine motor skills involved, for instance, in writing a w or a p, are too complicated for the child who cannot write on a straight line and who cannot make horizontal or vertical lines which are connected. Children learn manuscript writing in school before they learn cursive writing, on the theory that it correlates better with reading, and is, therefore, easier to learn. Most normal children can make the transition from manuscript to cursive writing easily when they are approximately eight or nine years old. The organically damaged child, who has already established the patterns of learning for manuscript writing, cannot make this transition, and the old skill which has already been learned prevents him from learning this new skill.

The child who has learned manuscript writing has learned to write in discrete forms, as there is no need to connect letters. In addition, the lines of direction are fairly consistent for each letter. Cursive writing, however, presents many problems. First, the letters have to be connected. Second, some single letters, like z, for instance, require at least five different directions of hand and eye movement within the letter.

The organically damaged child, however, can learn to write such letters as *m* and *u*, which have rounded forms and move horizontally across the page, much more easily than letters such as *i* and *t*, which require a retracing of the original line in an opposite direction. Letters such as *l*, *e*, and *g* are also difficult, because they require movements which are not parallel. One of the most common symptoms of diffuse organic malfunctioning may be the inability of a child to follow the directional lines along with the group in learning cursive writing.

The following three cases are typical examples of diffuse organic malfunctioning in childhood.

Helen R.: Female, Age 9, IQ 96

TEACHER'S DESCRIPTION OF BEHAVIOR

In the classroom, Helen is badly co-ordinated. The other children don't like to play group games with her at recess because she plays almost every game poorly—dropping the ball, not running fast enough, etc. She is very affectionate toward the teacher, attempting close physical contact whenever possible.

During classroom periods of quiet seat work, she is distracted very easily. She finds excuses to sharpen her pencils, to pull the blinds down because the light hurts her eyes, etc. She is constantly in movement, pulling at her shirt, twisting her legs, biting strands of her hair. She appears to be overly stimulated by the simplest activities of other children. If another child leaves her seat for a valid reason, Helen somehow manages to become involved.

In academic work, Helen manages to keep up with the rest of the class although she appears to be struggling to do so. Her reading is adequate, but she still has too many reversals of simple words which somehow she has not been able to master. She has great difficulty, however, with writing, and because she is so concerned with the mechanics of writing, her spelling suffers. That is, the efforts that should be expended in the spelling per se, are spent in the mechanics of writing. Her arithmetic is below fourth-grade level (second grade). Although she has the concepts of adding and subtracting, she has no memorized skills. Multiplication and division are completely beyond her comprehension.

PSYCHOLOGICAL REPORT

Helen was very eager and co-operative. She appeared to be most anxious to please the examiner, and throughout the examination such questions as, "Am I doing all right?" or, "Was that right?" were frequent. Even though she was reassured as much as possible by the examiner, she continued to ask for support. Thus, she gave a picture of feeling inadequate, helpless, and vulnerable to the testing situation.

On the Wechsler Intelligence Scale for Children, Helen obtained a verbal IQ of 111, a performance IQ of 85, and a full scale of 96. She had notable difficulty in tests of visual-motor co-ordination. This fact, coupled with the discrepancy between the verbal and the performance IQ's, tends toward suggesting some neurological involvement which is incapacitating her at this time.

This difficulty in motor co-ordination was also noted on the other projective tests. On the Figure Drawing Test, for instance, she had marked difficulty drawing a body that was in proportion to the head. There were obvious distortions of proportions as well as an inability to draw a unified figure. This, again, suggests a neurological involvement.

On the other projective material, Helen gave evidences of feeling inadequate and unsure of herself. This feeling of inadequacy, in part, appears to be related to her own concept of herself as a vague, undefinable person. She is not sure of her own role in relation to others. Her social relationships, therefore, while superficially good, are emotionally meaningless. Because she senses her own inadequacy, and because she is ready to assume the blame for it, she has become extremely anxious and guilt-ridden. She feels unconsciously that she must be at fault for what is wrong with her.

Summary. Because of her poor integrative performance on tests of visual motor co-ordination, and because she experiences feelings of inadequacy, helplessness, and hopelessness to an inordinate degree, it is felt that Helen's problem is essentially of an organic nature. A complete neurological examination is advised.

DEVELOPMENTAL HISTORY

Helen was a so-called "blue baby" at birth—a blood transfusion was required, and there were a few seconds when Helen appeared to have stopped breathing. Her early development was slow. She crawled at one year, walked at two and one-half years, talked only at three and one-half.

NEUROLOGICAL DIAGNOSIS

A neurological examination revealed that some very minor damage appeared to have occurred at birth, when apparently the brain had not had sufficient oxygen for those few seconds when breathing had either stopped or been excessively shallow.

David K.: Male, Age 13, IQ 101

TEACHER'S DESCRIPTION OF BEHAVIOR

When David was first admitted to class, he was unable to conform to any program, even the very elastic type of activity planned for him. He was impulsively aggressive toward both the children in the school and the teachers. He showed a great deal of stubbornness, and deliberate, vicious, derogatory invectives were part of his verbal behavior, indicating openly a great dislike for both people and school activities. He indulged in infantile temper tantrums, kicking and crying, and did not respond at all to coaxing or pressure until he had worn himself out and was ready to stop.

The results of untimed power achievement tests, given because they afford testing under the least amount of pressure, indicated that David's academic level ranges from sixth to eighth grade, averaging into about the seventh-grade level.

PSYCHOLOGICAL REPORT

David obtained an IQ of 92 on the Performance Section of the Wechsler Intelligence Scale for Children. On the Rorschach, David displayed inadequate figure-ground differentiation in his perceptual performance and uncritical generalization in his thinking. He also gave evidence of being unable to establish a meaningful relationship with another person. His phantasy was concerned with men who fly through the air. There was the absence of normal emotional responses. He was inclined, however, to sudden emotional outbursts which were irrational and lacking in apparent motivation. David also had auditory hallucinations in which he heard the voice of God and spirits talking to him. He had visual hallucinations; he saw dead people at night. He believed that he could hear for long distances and through walls, and that he could fly like Superman. The diagnosis made was chronic brain syndrome of unknown cause with psychosis.

DEVELOPMENTAL HISTORY

David was a full-term, normal baby who walked at one year and talked at fourteen months. The only serious illness in his childhood was spinal meningitis, for which he was hospitalized at the age of two and one-half years. There were no apparent difficulties until David started school at the age of six. He was hyperactive, destructive, and easily provoked into aggression. This has been his pattern ever since.

David's home is apparently a fairly adequate one. He lives in Staten Island with his mother, father, and a younger sister, eleven years old.

His mother is forty-eight years old, his father, fifty-one, and they have been maintaining a fairly normal home since the father's return from sixteen years of service in the army.

NEUROLOGICAL DIAGNOSIS

A neurological examination determined an abnormal electroencephalogram. Diagnosis: chronic brain syndrome.

Janet A.: Female, Age 9, IQ 94

TEACHER'S DESCRIPTION OF BEHAVIOR

She had consistent school failures and exhibited poor relationship to both children and adults. She had no attention span and no ability to concentrate. She was disruptive, hyperactive, and notably poor in many manual activities. Her reading was on a third-grade level; arithmetic, below first grade. She could do no cursive writing. Her spelling was on a third-grade level, providing she was given enough time to complete each word.

PSYCHOLOGICAL REPORT

The Rorschach indicated poor perceptual levels, and perseveration. The examiner noted a complete feeling of helplessness and a need for reassurance. On the Stanford-Binet, Form L, she scored an IQ of 94, showing, however, definite discrepancies between performance items and verbal items. Her perception was poor; she gave primitive forms. On the Bender-Gestalt Visual Motor Test, her maturational level was approximately at the sixth year. Her figure drawing was out of proportion, indicating immaturity and imbalance in body image.

DEVELOPMENTAL HISTORY

Her mother's pregnancy was normal until a virus infection in the ninth month. Birth was difficult. Maturation was within normal limits —talking at one and one-half years, walking at two years, and toilet training completed at two and one-half years. The only evidence of difficulty was poor co-ordination in play.

NEUROLOGICAL DIAGNOSIS

There were no discernible brain lesions, but an abnormal electro-encephalogram suggested diffuse organic malfunctioning.

SUMMARY

The child with a mild organic disturbance often cannot be differentiated from the schizophrenic or neurotic child. While there is no gross

organic malfunctioning, distractible behavior, bizarre thinking, instability, and overaggressiveness can be traced to minor neurological ab-
normalities. Such children can often be detected in the classroom because they present specific learning problems. One of their most obvious
difficulties in learning is their inability to transfer from manuscript to
cursive writing. For teaching cursive writing, therefore, special methods
have to be evolved, directed specifically toward overcoming the effects
of the organic abnormality.

Chapter IV

The Neuroses

All psychotic individuals are considered to be disturbed, but all disturbed individuals are certainly not psychotic. It is apparent that there can be many shades of disturbance between extreme psychotic deviation and normal acceptable behavior. These disturbances vary in degree and severity, depending largely upon variations in causative factors and individual differences.

The term *neurosis* should not be thought of as a label for a particular disease entity, but rather as a diagnostic indicator describing a certain range of severity in maladjustment. Neurosis is considered to be milder in degree than psychosis, insofar as neurotic disorders are not characterized by removal from reality. In differentiating psychosis from neurosis by a simple definition, the distinguishing factor in psychosis may be described as a break with reality while in neurosis there is no denial of the existence of reality, merely an attempt to cope with the pain of it through the formation of pathological symptomatology. The neurotic child is so traumatized, both by experiences which cause him anxiety and by the unacceptability of his impulses, that he handles the experiences ineptly while at the same time struggling to repress his impulses into the unconscious.

The Role of the Unconscious

The concept of the unconscious was first formulated by Freud in his psychoanalytic system of psychology. This concept is widely used today in almost all schools of psychology, even those that basically disagree with Freud's other tenets. The term *unconscious* is frequently synonymous with the term *subconscious*. Both refer to the dynamic processes operating below the level of awareness. Degrees of awareness can vary from processes upon which attention is acutely focused to those which are completely below the level of consciousness and which sometimes cannot, under any circumstances, be brought to a conscious level. When a child is reading, for example, he is most acutely aware of the material being read, less aware of the peripheral environment and not at all aware, perhaps, of the anxiety which may be engendered by some of the content of the reading material.

Human functioning which is below the level of consciousness is thought to center in basic instinctual drives which constantly seek satisfaction, like self-preservation, hunger, and sex. There are various concepts of the nature of these drives and much disagreement as to the exact definition of their source. Freud explains them as biological impulses which are by nature primitive, unmoral, unorganized, and illogical, constantly striving for supremacy in the individual and influencing all behavior. On the other hand, some authorities conceive of drives in somewhat broader terms, including not only the basic biological instincts, but also the more superficial wishes and desires apparent in everyday experiences. Warren's *Dictionary of Psychological Terms* defines drives as "any intra-organic activity or condition which supplies stimulation for a particular type of behavior. It covers both organic activating conditions, such as hunger, and presumably also cerebral conditions, such as mental set or such as desire for a particular object."

For our purposes, however, a drive is considered to be any unconscious, satisfaction-demanding force, whether it be nutritional, self-preservative, sexual, or aggressive. Clinical observation has indicated that, whatever the nature of drives, their control is based upon the use of the various defense mechanisms which force these drives into the unconscious. For example, it is normal in the process of development for a child to experience feelings of hostility and aggression toward his parents. Because a mother or father is an inhibiting agent who does not permit the child free expression of his desires, the child views the parent with some anger. The child, however, cannot permit himself to recognize his own anger because he also loves his parents and it creates intense guilt within him for him to be angry with them. The child therefore represses the anger, denying it even to himself. The anger is relegated into the area known as the unconscious because the child convinces himself that it does not exist.

DEFENSE MECHANISMS

A defense mechanism is a protective device which permits one to conceal an unacceptable truth from oneself. Instincts, particularly in childhood, are continually in stormy conflict with acceptable, normal, ethical judgment. A child is constantly attempting to develop and utilize his defense mechanisms while trying to adjust to an ever changing environment. Although it would be an impossible task to describe all the various forms of this adjustment that even one person uses in attempting to function adequately, the science of behavior has clarified certain specific defense mechanisms which are fairly commonly labeled and which can, therefore, be useful as a point of reference. These mechanisms are evident in the behavior of all people. When they are adequate, they are valuable in explaining normal behavior, and when they are exaggerated, they can be seen as a basis for disturbed behavior. Since all defense mechanisms are used to control primitive impulses, and because defenses are so closely intertwined behaviorally, they often cannot be clearly differentiated.

Defenses function on an unconscious level. The individual is not aware of his *modus operandi,* nor does he consciously decide to use any particular defense. To a large extent, defense mechanisms may be viewed as the habitual way in which an individual has learned to respond to situations and the emotional manner in which he handles life experiences. These defenses may be categorized into the following classifications: compensation, rationalization, regression, repression, and sublimation. An understanding of defense mechanisms is essential to the clarification and evaluation of both normal and disturbed personality patterning, particularly in relation to the neuroses.

Compensation. One of the most common mechanisms of adjustment is compensation. Compensation implies an unconscious resistance against the threat of failure or a feeling of inferiority, whether physical, intellectual, or social. All people, however, do not necessarily compensate in defending against their inadequacies. The utilization of compensation as a defense mechanism is dependent 1) upon the individual seeing himself as inadequate, and 2) upon the degree of facility he has developed in order to overcome this feeling of inadequacy.

Compensation results in an emphasis on a particular personality characteristic or a substitution of a different characteristic in order to conceal the deficiency that the individual feels is present. One child who has a speech defect may unconsciously compensate for this defect, overcoming the frustration associated with it by fighting it and becoming an actor with perfect diction. Another child with the same defect will strive, perhaps, for excellence in an area where speech is not essential, such as becoming an outstanding athlete. In the first case there is an emphasis on the original deficiency and a mastery of it, whereas in the second case, the substitution of a completely different characteristic made the child feel adequate in a new and different situation. In both of these cases there was unconscious compensation, and an adequate adjustment was the result.

Sometimes, however, the inadequacy a child experiences may not have its roots in actuality; instead, it is the result of his own irrational emotionality. The child may feel inadequate because to him alone, his nose appears to be too large and ugly. This feeling about his nose, which the analysts would describe as displacement of the feelings of inadequacy actually centered on his penis, would obviously have no basis in reality. A nose, however, is a more acceptable part of the anatomy to talk about than the penis. The child, therefore, reacts to the believed deficiency of his nose as if it were an obvious, realistic one, and could, as a result, develop compensatory behavior with respect to an inferiority which actually does not exist. This child may overcompensate for his chosen deficit by referring to his nose frequently, perhaps becoming a wit, as in *Cyrano de Bergerac* where much of the humor is centered about the nose. The importance of any inferiority or inadequacy experienced by the child, is not that he actually *is* inferior or inadequate, but that he *feels* inferior or inadequate.

Children are dependent, small in stature, lacking in strength, and constantly frustrated by these inadequacies as well as by the demands made upon them by adults. Frequently these lacks are compensated for in noisy behavior, aggressive play, fighting, teasing, or other outgoing activities permitted, primarily, only when children are with their peers. Children also use compensation in another type of substitution. For example, being overly unselfish may hide a fear of being selfish; being overly good may hide the fear of being bad; or being overtyrannical may hide the fear of being incompetent. When for some reason a child is afraid to assert himself in the usual acceptable ways, yet feels a great need to express his adequacy, he may resort to bullying, stealing, truanting, destroying property, or any number of other distorted forms of compensatory behavior. Such extremes in conduct are likely to be unconscious compensations, momentarily satisfying for the child, but disturbing to others. Compensations which are socially unacceptable differ from normal compensatory behavior, not in the way in which the mechanism operates, but rather in an exaggeration in quality and degree of the resultant behavior. When there is excessive aggressive compensation, the child may thwart some other needs, such as his need for love; and risk, in addition, the possibility of retaliation for his behavior by adults. Moreover, in such cases the mechanism adopted is inadequate and does not reduce the anxiety and tension associated with the original need. The bullying child who overcompensates for his inadequacy and insecurity suffers the disapproval of adults, and does not achieve the kind of adequacy he is really seeking. Instead, the anxiety he had hoped to alleviate is actually intensified. Unacceptable behavior, operating under these conditions, wastes energy in misdirection, gives no return in real satisfaction, and unfortunately is likely to be expressed in continued extremes of conduct.

When, on the other hand, the extreme behavior is that of withdrawal rather than aggression, the compensatory mechanism is again being used unsatisfactorily. The child, in trying to relieve his tensions and anxieties, may completely withdraw from a situation and become lethargic, unresponsive, and uncommunicative. Extreme withdrawal is dangerous and may indicate a serious pathological disturbance, possibly even one culminating in psychosis.

Projection. Projection is the mechanism whereby the individual unconsciously attributes to other persons or to things the feelings that he himself experiences. Just as a projector is used to throw off a film image onto a screen, so does the term *projection* mean attributing to other people the emotions which the individual himself experiences. When the very young child cries and says, "Naughty table!" because he, himself, has bumped into it, he removes the onus of his activity from himself and puts it onto the table. What the child really feels is, "I am naughty," but this realization is too painful for him to make, and he displaces his responsibility upon another object. Projection, therefore, serves as a mechanism which permits the individual to relieve himself of the anxiety and responsibility associated with his own behavior. If, in hating someone and in feeling tremendous aggressive urges toward a specific person, the individual can believe that it isn't *he* who is doing the hating, but rather that the other person hates him, he is able to ease his own anxiety. Thus, his feelings of "I hate you" are converted into "you hate me." A person, therefore, who is afraid of his own aggressive impulses obtains some relief from his anxiety by attributing aggression to other people. Through the mechanism of projection, the individual changes the internal danger—the threatening feelings and emotions which cause him discomfort and anxiety—into an external danger which is, therefore, easier for him to accept.

Projection is a normal reaction pattern for all people at some time, and because it is generally agreed to be universal, a whole new field of psychological tests have arisen which uses the mechanism of projection as its rationale. These tests are known as projective devices. For example, a person is asked to invent a story about a picture which is presented to him, or perhaps he is given a piece of clay and asked merely to make something out of it. He might be given paints, crayons, or pencil, and asked to draw a picture. He could also be given a series of ink blots to look at, and be asked to express what real objects they look like to him. The individual delves into his own emotional resources and projects his feelings and attitudes upon the materials with which he is working. In this way, ten different people could tell ten different stories to the same picture, each revealing, in his own way, the attitudes, emotions, and conflicts which are characteristic of him. One child, for instance, may make a figure with a piece of clay, call it "daddy," and then destroy it by thumping furiously upon it. Another child may make the same figure, call it by the same name, and cradle it lovingly. Obviously, these two children are giving expression to the same stimulus with two very different basic responses. Yet, if they were to be asked verbally how they felt about their fathers, the chances of their being able to describe their underlying feelings in words would be indeed slim. Because projective tests permit the trained examiner an opportunity for minute observation of behavior concomitant to an expression of pent-up emotions, they are valuable techniques for use in personality evaluation.

Rationalization. Inadequacies can be defended not only by action, but also by thoughts and words. When a child justifies his unacceptable behavior by giving socially acceptable reasons for it, he is attempting to deny unconscious motives which he finds too painful to recognize, and to hide the truth from both himself and others. This pattern of behavior utilizes a defense mechanism called rationalization. Rationalization is a protective device which, like all defenses, is unconscious, and used to hide from oneself the presence of unacceptable impulses. It is a face-saving device used for self-justification and is a part of the everyday living of every person. Arithmetic examples are not completed because "my pencil broke." A woodworking project is poorly done because "the wrong tools were around." A game is lost because "the referee favored the other team." Children believe their rationalizations and they expect others to do the same. *They are not consciously lying.* For example, a boy who does not get to school on time might really believe that the reason for his tardiness was an inaccurate clock, although he knew the clock was wrong; or a need to wait for his brother, whom he, himself, delayed by teasing; or, perhaps, a late breakfast which he caused by making his mother waste time in waking him. He cannot accept the fact that the lateness was really caused by his reluctance to go to school. His instinct might have been of an aggressive nature, and his desire, perhaps, was to be a truant. Truancy is not accepted by parents or the school authorities, so he tries to stifle his true feelings, substituting lateness for truancy and establishing a reason for his lateness which he can consciously accept. He cannot admit the truth to himself so he "lies" to himself, as well as to others, consciously believing it to be completely true.

When the need for success and the fear of failure is overpowering, rationalization may be exaggerated, and in that case could assume proportions approaching delusions. It can interfere with logical thought to the extent that a child can deceive himself with even less than half a truth. The adolescent drug addict, for example, may rationalize his addiction to drugs by explaining that he needs a "lift" when he is tired, or that his mother recently died, or that he worries about school, etc., ad infinitum, finding it more confortable to believe any or all of these reasons rather than the truth, which could be anything from an unconscious death wish directed against the father to an unconscious fear of homosexuality. In his anxiety he is making an attempt to justify, to himself and to others, an unacceptable act by means of half-plausible, half-fantastic logic.

Rationalization should be carefully examined and must not be confused with conscious lying. The child who lies is conscious of the lie, which he wants others to believe. Rationalization is an unconscious lie with which the child deceives himself. The child who consciously lies, for instance, may deny hitting another child, saying that he didn't do it. The child who rationalizes may say he hit the other child because "he hit me first," unaware that he deliberately provoked the attack. In both cases, the motivation of impulsive aggression is present. The lying child denies the act, knowing his denial to be a lie, whereas the child who rationalizes does not deny the aggression, but deceives himself into believing that the aggression was justified and that the blame rests on another.

Regression. Another adjustive mechanism used to escape from difficulty is a reversion to primitive or infantile modes of behavior. This defense is called regression, and represents an unconscious retreat from the anxiety of distressing situations to patterns of behavior which brought satisfaction at an earlier stage of development. In a broad sense, regression is inherent in all forms of defense mechanisms as well as in many types of serious maladjustments.

The most obvious manifestations of regression are seen in the behavior of young children, who, when thwarted, tend to respond to a situation on an infantile level. A three-year-old who at the birth of a sibling loses the attention of his parents, may revert to crawling, thumb-sucking, or need spoon-feeding and care just like an infant. The adolescent who throws his notebook in the basket after failing a test, or kicks a chair over, is exhibiting momentary regressive behavior. Regression, then, is the return to a relatively simple, crude, early-life mode of response based upon earlier satisfaction patterns. It is an avoidance mechanism employed in an attempt to evade the necessity for making a realistic adjustment.

Regressions usually occur at particular moments of stress in the life experience of an individual. A six-year-old who is faced with the death of a beloved grandparent may suddenly begin to cling to his parents and demand to be hugged and caressed by them. He may also become enuretic at night. This reaction, of course, must be viewed in the light of the real situation which caused the child to suffer emotional trauma. He may cling to his parents in order to make sure that they too won't be taken away from him. In acting like a baby, therefore, he gains for himself the security he experienced in infancy, a period in his life when he was completely safe. Regressions, therefore, regardless of the age at which they occur, are always indicative of an individual's wish to return to a previous stage of development in which he felt complete safety and security.

Temporary regressions are fairly normal in childhood. As an individual matures into adult life, however, he should not find it necessary to regress into childish forms of behavior even though he encounters a particular emotional crisis. A mature adult should have developed enough inner resources to cope with difficulties in a manner commensurate with his level of maturity, without needing to resort to regressive forms of behavior.

Regression can be a part of normal behavior when it is used as a diverting activity like recreation or relaxation from the daily monotonies of living, or as an emotional safety valve in times of stress. Boisterous behavior at a party, childlike enthusiasm for a sport, or childish weeping at a time of bereavement are beneficial regressions which relieve temporary strain. In a large measure, however, regressions in the behavior patterns of both adults and children are indicative of personality disorders and are seriously injurious when they become habitual. The emotional immaturity exhibited in regressive behavior is characteristic of many severe neurotic and psychotic disturbances. The child who sucks his thumb at the age of fourteen, the bed-wetter at the age of ten, the child who has temper tantrums at fifteen, are all giving evidence of behavior which netted satisfaction at a previous level of development, but which are inappropriate to their present age level. They are exhibiting regressive behavior.

Repression and Denial. Impulses that are in conflict with social values, and primitive, selfish urges that run counter to the code of society, can be overwhelming and anxiety provoking. Satisfying these impulses is out of the question. In fact, even giving thought to them causes feelings of guilt and greater anxiety. The child who inhibits the responses to these needs to the point of keeping himself from remembering their existence is using the mechanism of repression. Repression does not remove the instinctual drives. It merely permits the child to keep them from being recognized; consequently, there is no need for them to be satisfied. The most common form of repression, therefore, is forgetting.

Forgetting is generally selective in that the individual unconsciously wishes to forget a specific event or memory. Thus, most people forget the unpleasant incidents of life. A child quickly forgets that at first he did not like the new baby, or an adult forgets the address of someone whom he does not want to visit. Such forgetting is not merely coincidental; rather, it is actually a mechanism of behavior by which people repress the painful or unpleasant to such an extent that they are no longer aware of it.

From early infancy, a child is constantly required to restrain his desires when they are in conflict with the wishes of adults. The child is required to learn that inclinations which are disapproved of socially must be suppressed. A child's early aggressive behavior, for instance, meets with censure from adults. The child, then, in order to gain the approval of adults, suppresses his primitive destructive urges and inhibits his activities. When the fear of a drive becomes so strong that inhibition and suppression act to force its disappearance into the unconscious, so that there is no longer any apparent knowledge of the existence of the drive, this is the phenomenon known as repression.

The repression of undesirable tendencies, of course, is good, necessary, and an inherent part of the normal process of maturation. One of the ways to adjust to a conflict situation is by inhibiting undesirable impulses and by repressing them into the unconscious. There is always the possibility, however, that these impulses might somehow intrude momentarily into consciousness. Everyday slips of the tongue are examples of repression in which some certain previously inhibited, unacceptable thought comes to light in a somewhat unexpected manner. A child may invite another child to his birthday party by saying, "Come to my present, no, I mean, party." This child is trying to handle the relationship between party and present in an adult, acceptable fashion. He is really thinking, "Give me a present." In this example, the child has learned that being selfish is unacceptable and meets with disapproval. He therefore suppresses the selfish wish, repressing it into the unconscious, but the repression is not completely successful in that it emerges from the unconscious in a slip of the tongue. Similarly, an adult reading art criticism which states that in a particular painting "the woman was brilliantly expressed," may misread the sentence as "the woman was brilliantly exposed." Thus, he gives an indication of underlying sexual impulses which were, to a large extent, suppressed until that moment.

Repression does not mean that the unacceptable impulses lie dormant or disappear. When impulses are unconsciously forgotten, they may continue to rankle in the unconscious. Unless a substitute satisfaction can be found for them, deviate functioning may result. The destructive child who successfully represses his destructive impulses may substitute leadership qualities and thus satisfy his aggressive needs. When repression is not successful, however, and there is no adequate acceptable substitute to satisfy unacceptable impulses, the child may either withdraw completely and be afraid to act, or he may lose his conscious control and act out the primitive drives. The result of unsuccessful repression is continuous tension, blocking, anxiety, volcanic outbursts, or antisocial behavior.

Repression, then, may sometimes control the expression of conscious conflict at the risk of engendering precarious unconscious turmoil. When this unconscious conflict is severe, it may find outlet in anomolies of behavior and neurotic symptoms, seriously interfering with adaptive behavior. Repression, as a defense mechanism, is at best a method of controlling unacceptable feelings. When extreme repression gives way under stress, however, the result may be hallucinations, delusions, or a complete lack of emotional control.

Denial mechanisms are closely related to repression. By denying a situation or a drive or a conflict, the individual unconsciously refuses to admit that it exists. Thus, there are some individuals who refuse to take out life insurance, and in denying themselves of insurance, unconsciously feel they cannot die. Similarly, other persons refuse to attend funeral services or see a physician. Thus, they deny death or illness. If they don't "face" a situation, they cannot believe it will happen.

Simple denial is a primitive mechanism, most frequently manifested by children. "You are *not* my Daddy," when the child is angered by the parent, is a common denial mechanism. It is the child's way of being omnipotent and believing in the efficacy of the magical wish. In children, this mechanism is acceptable. In adults, it is an expression of an immature level of functioning, representing a magical wish-fulfillment stage of development in childhood. With maturity, of course, feelings of omnipotence are relinquished, and with them, the mechanism of denial as a prime method of adjustive behavior.

With maturity, the gradual knowledge and acceptance of reality makes this defense impossible. Thus, it is clearly a defense found most often in children, in neurotics whose other defenses have become inadequate, or in psychotics whose hold on reality is a tenuous one. Denial, however, is not pathological when it is expressed in the form of daydreams by normal adults or children. Thus, in phantasy, adults as well as children may deny an unpleasant fact by the substitution of a wish.

Sublimation. Sublimation is the channeling of unacceptable impulses into socially acceptable behavior, by substituting for an unacceptable drive one which is appropriate for relieving the original drive and which has, at the same time, a socially desirable aspect. Examples of sublimation can be found in the behavior of all people. It is seen in the substitution of highly approved forms of activity for disapproved selfish desires; primitive urges are redirected into acceptable, useful behavior patterns. Sublimation is the unconscious transformation of instinctual drives into useful goals, an emotional process which, if successful, makes for the re-integration of the personality on a higher level.

The process of sublimation should be of utmost interest to the teacher as a tool for the control of the antisocial impulses and desires manifested by disturbed children. It is a valuable technique for adjusting the child's inner drives to the demands of the environment. The domineering bully can be helped to use his strength and his need for self-assertion in leadership activities which bring him approval and with which he can succeed. In the same way, vigorous participation in recreational activities can be encouraged as a means of sublimating aggressive impulses, thereby circumventing delinquent behavior. Sexual sublimation, which is essential in our society, can also be instrumental in directing energy toward constructive, purposeful activity, both physical and mental, by stimulating interest in sports, avocations, social activities, or intellectual labors. The use of sublimation affords the child satisfaction, while permitting him to reduce his anxiety at the same time. It also affords him an opportunity to function adequately in society in a manner which is acceptable to himself and which is worthy of approval by others.

According to Fenichel the normal individual has successful defenses in that he has the capacity to sublimate his instinctual drives.[1] Sublimation is characterized by the rerouting of the instinctual drives from direct expression to indirect discharge in a more socially acceptable manner. With this mechanism functioning, a child can gratify his drives, lessen his anxiety, and thereby reduce the conflict between his instinctual demands and the dictates of his conscience. Sublimation is successful when a change of goal or an inhibition of aim is directed toward adequate acceptable behavior.

REACTION FORMATION

Reaction formations appear as characteristic of a certain form of repression. It can be described as a repression which not only masks or denies an unacceptable impulse, but at the same time tries to prove that exactly the opposite feeling exists. For example, an individual whose instinctual needs can be satisfied by dirt and disorder, but who finds this mode of living undesirable, handles his problem by developing opposite traits. He does a complete about-face and becomes compulsively orderly and neat. In like manner, a mother who is essentially hostile to her child, becomes overprotective; an individual who feels overstrong sexual and antimoral impulses becomes a fanatic reformer, or a moral crusader. All of these are examples of reactive formations.

Frequently it is difficult to determine the differences between sublimation and reaction formations. To clarify the difference, one may say that in sublimation, the original impulse is channelized into a more acceptable direction, but the original drive remains essentially the same. A person with destructive, sadistic impulses sublimates them and satisfies himself by becoming a surgeon instead of a criminal. The social outcome may differ, but the original drive is unchanged. In reactive formation, the original drive is suppressed, or repressed, and there is no discharge of the original impulse. Thus, the moral crusader never does release his original destructive impulses. Instead, he subsitutes for it behavior that merely goes in the opposite direction. Persons who

---

[1] O. Fenichel, *The Psychoanalytic Theory of Neurosis* (New York: W. W. Norton and Company, 1945), pp. 141–43.

habitually adopt such mechanisms, therefore, may be considered repressed individuals. Their repressions cause great anxiety because there is no appropriate release of the instinctual drive. To summarize the difference briefly, in sublimation the original impulse is expressed and its energy is withdrawn in favor of its substitute. In reaction formation, the original impulse is held in check without finding discharge.

SYMPTOM DEVELOPMENT

There are no sharp lines of demarcation between the various forms of defense mechanisms. Reaction formation is related to repression, repression to sublimation, sublimation to reaction formation, reaction formation to denial, denial to repression, repression to projection, and so forth in a circle.

The defense mechanisms work to avoid the full expression of primitive instinctual drives, which are in conflict with expected, accepted modes of behavior. When there is great difficulty in reconciling these primitive strivings with the external code of behavior demanded by society, tension and anxiety are the results. A child, for instance, is always trying to adjust to the demands of reality which he knows exist, and which he knows he must meet. The child normally has a need to gratify his drive for aggression, but it is equally as normal for that same child to feel the need to curb this aggression. The conflict between the drive to assert aggression, on the one hand, and the need to conform, on the other, somehow must be resolved. The normal child may resolve it by means of defense mechanisms which help him meet the demands of the environment while permitting him to divert his aggression and express it through socially acceptable behavior.

The neurotic child, on the other hand, is unsuccessful in his attempts to maintain a good balance between the satisfaction of a drive and the need to meet the demands of social conformity; consequently, he adopts a form of behavior which may be considered maladjusted. When the unconscious inner impulse is one with which the neurotic child cannot live, when it is antagonistic to his concepts of morality or ethics, when it is unacceptable to his conscience, he denies expression to this drive without being able to employ acceptable defenses. He does, however, substitute for it a behavior pattern which, although realistically unsatisfactory, is more acceptable to him than the recognition of the original unacceptable impulse.

The neurotic child, then, employs defense mechanisms with which he attempts to relieve anxiety, but the defense mechanisms fail. In this sense, the defense mechanisms become sick and a symptom is formed to act as an additional defense and help the child control the drives he views as unacceptable. The child maintains the neurotic symptoms after they are no longer useful and continues to function inadequately, suffering great emotional anxiety. According to Halpern:

"In the healthy individual, the defenses he musters when anxiety threatens operate well enough to reduce or allay that anxiety. There is no need for the continued emphasis on certain mechanisms. However, where the defenses do not operate successfully, there is a continual compulsive need for them and they are invoked even when the immediate situation does not demand their presence and activity." [2]

A child who develops a neurosis has changed his mode of behavior so that he will be protected not only when he is faced with danger, but as if that danger were continuously present. For example, a child who develops gastrointestinal upset preceding a particularly important school examination, such as a final term test or school entrance examination, is facing a real anxiety-provoking situation, and develops a physical symptom which passes as soon as the trauma of the actual situation is passed. The child may also develop diarrhea before the test and then rationalize his possible failure by blaming his physical condition at the time he was taking the test. This type of symptom, or a similar neurotic pattern formation, dependent upon the personality involved, is a normal reaction to a terrifying situation. It is only when the reaction of gastrointestinal disturbance becomes chronic, and appears even when there is no real anxiety-provoking situation, that it may be considered a form of neurosis. The anxiety then exists in the

---

[2] F. Halpern, *A Clinical Approach to Children's Rorschach* (New York: Grune and Stratton, 1953), p. 59.

child, and the child reacts as though the traumatic situation were constantly present.

Children have to reconcile their primitive, unacceptable impulses
with the demands of the environment in a way that leaves them satisfied while permitting acceptable behavior. A child who is inadequate
in his ability to find equilibrium acts as if he does not know what is
acceptable to the environment, and he becames anxious. In order to
alleviate this anxiety, he develops pathological symptoms which are
indicative of neurosis. Neurotic symptomatology falls into certain broad
categories, generally described under such diagnostic labels as anxiety
neurosis, hysterical conversions, phobias, and obsessive compulsions.
It is unusual, however, to find a disturbance limited to one specific
neurotic symptom or a particular character trait. The child who is an
obsessive-compulsive may also be phobic; the child who has a tic generally also suffers from overwhelming anxiety.

All neurotic symptoms stem from the repression of instinctual drives.
When the normal defense mechanisms fail to operate successfully, the
individual must alleviate the anxiety engendered by this failure by
adopting distorted forms of reactions. Thus, the neuroses are "sick"
reactions to the basic defenses which have failed the individual.

Anxiety Neurosis. All defense mechanisms, whether normal inhibitory restrictions of a function, or unusual deviations resulting in
pathological symptomatology, are related to anxiety. Anxiety, as a common symptom of neurotic functioning, however, not only accompanies
symptom development, but is a symptom in and of itself when it assumes a distorted, unrealistic, disproportionate form of expression. It is
the result of constantly expected inner danger with a feeling of abject
helplessness in the face of an anticipated threat. Continuous doubts,
tensions, and frustrations leave the child in a precarious state of threat
from disrupting inner and outer forces. This free-floating form of
anxiety is not attached to any ideational content and does not have any
adequate defenses to circumvent it. Children who are anxiety-ridden
experience deep-seated feelings of inadequacy, and a sense of insecurity
which causes unhappiness without compensation in the usual pleasures

of childhood. The anxiety seems to be unmotivated, or without any apparent reason, or is precipitated by trivial occurrences. The child lives with a fear of impending calamity, and in a state of anticipatory anxiety which serves no function and from which there is no flight. This type of free-floating anxiety arises as a response to internal strivings which are unacceptable to the child. Teachers have many opportunities for observing this type of behavior since it is so pervasive that it colors all areas of functioning. It is not uncommon among teachers to describe certain children as "nervous" and "high-strung." This type of child seems to be easily upset, jittery, and gives a diffuse feeling of being ill at ease. There seems to be nothing specific that can be easily labeled, but there is a general awareness of discomfort. These children may be very concerned about their own status and may try too hard to do well. They never seem to enjoy fully any success they may achieve, because they are continuously dissatisfied with the results of their own efforts. Anxiety pervades all their activities and is all-consuming of their energies. When a disturbed child is anxious, his anxiety goes beyond the realm of rational fear. It is focused upon unimportant details and on unrelated material, and emphasizes areas not usually associated with the need to be anxious. There seems to be a constant dissatisfaction, a constant probing, and a continual searching for something undefined and elusive. This symptom is differentiated from normal fear and anxiety in that it is not related to actual conditions. Naturally, a certain amount of anxiety in response to a real anxiety-provoking situation is normal. When a child faces, for example, a performance on stage, anxiety is realistic, and part of the normal emotional pattern of most children facing a similar situation. When, however, anxiety is directed toward everyday routines, and is evident every time a child has to write lessons in his notebook or each time his group lines up to go home, it is not realistic, and stems not from the external threat in the environment, but rather from the child's own inner promptings. These children may seek constant assurance and frequent support from the adults in the environment. Even though an activity is one in which the child has engaged every day, he looks for support over and over again. He asks for approval when drawing, for example, by asking the teacher to suggest a color to use. When he uses the suggested color, however, he again has to be reassured that it is correct. He constantly seeks direction and needs reassurance for all activities. He is unable to rely upon himself; yet, he is dissatisfied and uneasy even with reassurance. The anxious child is ambivalent. He cannot make up his mind. He gives up hope in favor of inactivity, trying in this way to relieve his torturing ambiguity. Anxiety can interfere with intellectual functioning, judgment, and emotional stability, and distort the individual's entire personality pattern.

The following production was elicited from a sixteen-year-old girl who was in a state of severe anxiety, and who was being observed in a psychiatric hospital. She was apathetic and had developed a completely hopeless outlook on life. Nevertheless, she was seeking reassurance through religion in the hope that her anxiety would be alleviated.

"If I wasn't such a coward and had faced life squarely in the face instead of trying to run away from it, I wouldn't be here. Life is too confusing. God gives you something that you learn to love and then He takes it back from you. Is that fair? When you go to church and ask God to help someone and He doesn't help them, but makes them worse, then what is the sense of going to church? But you've got to go to church. Laws were made by men. They are also broken by men. What does God have to do with that? I'm waiting quietly and patiently to go back home and try to live life the way it is supposed to be lived. I want to believe that God is good."

The overwhelming ambivalence which is evidenced engenders anxiety. First she expresses belief in God, then she gives reasons for her disbelief. She believes in man-made laws and then questions them. This inability to make up her mind pervades all her thinking, produces more anxiety, and consequently she is in a continuous state of inner tension.

Free-floating anxiety is the most common neurotic symptom. Frequently, as soon as the individual appears to develop some resources to overcome the anxiety it either dissipates or becomes elaborated into some external nonfocal behavior mannerism. Children often indicate anxiety through excessive and exaggerated motor functioning. Facial and body mannerisms, like constant movement of fingers or toes, continuous sucking in of saliva through the teeth, consistent gulping and hissing, or undirected impulsive motor activity, all of psychogenic origin, are expressions of the child's attempt to alleviate anxiety.

The child who has mannerisms is not aware of the movements he is making. He performs these activities in a habitual way, making them as much a part of his personality as the rhythm of his walk. The child who engages in manneristic motor movements either is constantly moving his extremities in quick, darting, tense motions, or is posturing his body, inclining his head to odd angulations, or indulging in distorted facial expressions. Mannerisms can be brought into the awareness of the child so that he can control his movements in the same way that a child can control a habit. For instance, if a teacher tells the child to stop kicking his toes, the child is capable of ceasing this activity for as long a time as he remains acutely aware of the kicking. As soon as the child loses the awareness of the mannerism, however—when he is not consciously controlling his activity—the mannerism reappears without his conscious knowledge. Mannerisms may be greatly apparent at some times and subside into oblivion at others. They are intensified by stress situations and alleviated in periods of relative calm.

Constant movement uses up unacceptable instinctual energies and alleviates the constriction of the anxious person, thereby dissipating the anxiety to some degree. Excessive motor activity which seems meaningless and undirected is an overt indicator of the anxiety which is taking hold of the child, and which he is trying to alleviate through movement. Physical symptomatology related to neurosis is varied and almost without end. It ranges from simple discomforts like frequent urination to serious malfunctioning like hysterical paralysis.

Conversion Hysteria. Conversion hysteria is the transformation of anxiety into bodily symptoms similar to actual physical illness. Hysteria is one of the most baffling of the neuroses in that its manifestations are so numerous. There is hardly a characteristic of true physical illness that cannot be reproduced by hysterical symptoms. The conversion hysteria symptoms relieve emotional tension and anxiety through physical changes. These changes include paralysis of all voluntary musculature and sensory systems, as well as autonomic smooth muscle dysfunction. All hysterical conversions are without any real physical foundation. The physical mechanisms which fall into dysfunction are actually able to function adequately. There is no organic basis for the disability, but the disability is as crippling to the person suffering from it as any organic disease. It is an attempt, although feeble and ineffectual, at a kind of adjustment. Conversion hysteria is a response to an anxiety-producing situation by which the individual transforms his unconscious impulses and the concomitant guilt associated with these drives into physiological dysfunction. The symptoms may be motor, sensory, or mental, and include such things as psychological fatigue, paralysis, blindness, deafness, tremors, tics, mutism, vomiting, amnesia, delirium, etc. It has become common knowledge that in wartime there is a prevalence of hysterical conversions. The soldier who wants to flee from battle is not able to do so both by his own conscience and by fear of retaliation from authority. His emotional conflict is tremendous and he is overwhelmed by anxiety. One morning he awakens to find that he cannot get out of bed. He tries, but he is paralyzed and he cannot move. Medical examination finds nothing wrong physically. The paralysis, then, is the symptom developed by the soldier through the repression of his desire to run from danger. It is a kind of wish fulfillment. Physical disability saves him from the disgrace of cowardice, justifies his removal from battle, and protects him from danger; simultaneously it satisfies his need of punishment for leaving his friends to possible harm in a way that, as far as he can see, arose through no fault of his own. Psychological study indicates that those who tend toward hysterical conversion are handling their anxiety in a childlike, dependent fashion which gets attention successfully while diverting both from themselves and from others their real motives.

Children who manifest gross unmanageable hysterical symptoms are fairly rare, although the numbers increase in adolescence. There are, however, many forms of motor activity prevalent in children which do fall into this category. Of particular importance are tics—the inappropriate, fleeting spasms of small muscles resulting in involuntary movements such as eye-blinking, grimacing, tongue-clicking, and head-jerking. Stammering, too, may be a form of tic in some cases. These symptoms, found to relieve anxiety at the time of a particular traumatic experience, are used as defenses in any anxiety-producing situations, regardless of the appropriateness of the defense. For example, a child who is witness to a terrible automobile accident may blink his eyes in an attempt to deny momentarily the unacceptable fear-producing situation. This blinking movement used to reduce his anxiety was originally initiated as a defense against a specific trauma, but continues to act as a defense in all other frightening, anxiety-producing situations.

The part of the body affected by the conversion depends, to a large extent, upon the particular repressed urge. A strong desire to look at something forbidden may result in hysterical blindness. The blind eye cannot look and this helps to keep repressed both the idea of looking and the wish to look. In the same way the child who is made to feel guilty about masturbating may attempt to repress his desires and allay his guilt by developing a debilitating hand spasm.

Hysteria, although more prevalent in adolescents and adults, is occasionally seen in young children, particularly the type of conversion related to one specific act. It may occur when the child finds it impossible to adjust to the immediate difficulties of life.

Ellen: Female, Age 11, IQ 140

Ellen was a "musical prodigy," excelling in an ability to play the piano. She had been studying for eight years when she began to complain that her arms felt funny and her little finger did not want to bend sometimes. Immediately preceding a concert at which she was to perform, all five fingers of the right hand became rigid and completely refused to bend, and the performance had to be cancelled. She was examined and nothing was found to be physically wrong with the hand. She could use it for writing, eating, or playing ball, but not for playing the piano. It was felt that this symptom was the result of a feeling of inadequacy aggravated by the threat of a more talented sibling and the pressures from an ambitious, dominating mother. The physical disability was apparently an unconscious escape from the need for competing with the sister, and alleviated the threat for failing to please the mother. It was also a punishment for the guilt associated with aggressive wishes against the mother.

Hysterical conversion can be either episodic, occurring at particular moments of stress, or it can be more permanent, continuing over long periods of time. Conversions are not forms of malingering. The child is not pretending to be ill; he actually *is* ill, even though the cause of the illness is not a physical one. An hysterical conversion is a regressive type of neurotic symptom which permits the child much dependency and affords him care and protection.

Phobias and Displacement Mechanisms. A phobia is an abnormal fear attached to a specific situation or object. The most prevalent phobias are fear of darkness, water, heights, crowds, open spaces, dirt, fire, and animals. Phobias represent the disguising of unconscious wishes, in which the anxiety relating to these wishes is displaced to a specific object or situation. The individual who develops a phobia recognizes the fear as illogical and unreasonable, but does not generally understand why he has the fear and feels helpless in overcoming it. Many normal people have minor phobias which do not really incapacitate them. A phobia, however, is considered neurotic when it is of much intensity, long duration, or interferes appreciably with ordinary daily activities. Many irrational fears can be traced to a specific terrifying forgotten event which occurred at some previous time.

This type of phobia is very amenable to treatment and usually disappears when its origin is brought into consciousness and its connection to a specific event clarified.

Janice S.: Female, Age 8, IQ 114

Janice was mortally afraid of vacuum cleaners. She went into temper tantrums every time she saw one. It was found that Janice, at the age of four, was in an accident while playing in the street and ran into the house with blood running from her nose to get the assistance of her mother. Her mother was vacuuming and the noise of the vacuum cleaner kept her mother from hearing her screams. Janice, who at that time thought she was bleeding to death, related the vacuum cleaner to neglect by her mother, and although she had no memory of this event, the irrational fear of vacuum cleaners persisted.

This type of phobia has a clear, logical origin; other phobias, more severe and disabling, are merely symbolic of the real cause of the fear. For example, one individual who has a fear of small enclosed places may have developed this fear as the result of being trapped in a box as an infant. Another child may evidence the same phobia, but in this case it may be a displaced fear of death. The phobia in the second child represents repressed unconscious guilt with its emotional tone displaced and shifted to an apparently harmless idea—the fear of enclosed places.

Phobias, which are the result of traumatic experiences based on an actual fear situation in the past, are easier to overcome than phobias which are the result of displacement. Fear of subways, for instance, may be the result of a displaced fear in relationship to a repressed drive. It is normal for the adolescent, for instance, to need satisfaction of a sexual drive. The normal adolescent girl controls her sexual impulses by deriving satisfaction from socially acceptable patterns of behavior, like flirting, dancing, dating, and indulging in those other forms of heterosexual relations which are inherent in the prevailing culture. This pattern of behavior whereby the individual uses acceptable defensive substitute behavior to help satisfy the original sexual drive is normal. In this way the individual relieves the anxiety connected with the drive. However, the neurotic adolescent girl who fears the strength of her sexual drives is unable to utilize the normal defenses like flirting, dating, etc., and must repress this drive to the point of not being consciously aware of it. The ungratified drive, which is repressed, causes anxiety which is unresolved and results in a displacement of this drive with a symptom that is feared less than the drive itself. Taking this concept to its logical conclusion, it could be stated that an adolescent who seeks sexual gratification is exhibiting normal defenses when she flirts in the subway. She is neurotic, however, when she refuses to go into the subway, using this irrational fear of subways as a means of repressing her sexual drives. In the latter case, her normal defense is not adequate. In order to cope with her anxiety, therefore, she develops a symptom—a phobia of subways—thus shifting her emotional investment to a harmless external object. In this way, she is attempting to hide from both herself and the world the nature of her sexual drive. Phobic reactions may appear as early as the second year of life. In children, they are frequently associated with a feeling of a lack of maternal protection and the unconscious frustrated aggressive wishes toward the mother. The phobia arises as a defense against anxiety which results from the repressed hostility. It is indicative of a state of abnormal anxiety which is clearly circumscribed, and which is frequently bound to some particular situation.

Obsessive Compulsions. An obsession is an idea which occurs repeatedly to the individual without an apparent external stimulus or cause. It is consciously recognized by the individual as unreasonable, painful, objectionable, inappropriate, etc., but there seems to be no escape. A compulsion is the motor counterpart of the obsession which impels the individual into action. Most persons can remember mild childish compulsive acts such as touching every lamp post, stepping on every crack in the sidewalk, repeating addresses of houses on the street, or counting steps. In these cases, the obsession precedes the compulsion in the form of a need to step on cracks, touch lamp posts, etc.; the compulsion is the motor activity involved, the actual acting-out of the idea.

Many people have counting compulsions, such as counting lights in theaters, bald-headed men in the orchestra, buttons on clothing, houses, trees, or anything else countable. Still others make certain compulsive movements like twisting hair while reading or running hands through hair while talking. Examples like these could be enumerated at great length in the process of describing commonly seen behavior which is still certainly within the limits of normal functioning.

These "normal" compulsions are akin to "bad" habits. They are usually related to specific situations, and are not incapacitating because they can be denied. They do not evolve into the type of obsession which is an all inclusive idea which pervades all behavior, nor is there a disabling anxiety directly connected with it.

All people are concerned with very special ideas or problems at particular periods in their life. The boy who is entering college can think of little else except college life. The girl who is preparing for her first date is excessively concerned with plans of what she will wear. The man who is without a job will be tremendously worried about how he will support his family. Ideas like these may temporarily overwhelm a person, but they are not considered to be obsessions. They are merely problems which have to be solved; when the solution is found, they cease to be the individual's prime and exclusive thought. The individual will be able, upon solution of the problem, to free himself from the persistence of the idea, and return to more spontaneous and flexible thinking patterns. The obsessed person, however, cannot free himself from his obsession because it is based only partially on a reality situation and because the individual does not know why the idea presents itself. Sometimes the individual may recognize the obsession to be foolish, but he nevertheless cannot control it. For instance, an obsessed person may feel that he has to touch doorknobs. So he will touch every doorknob he sees. The obsession might grow so that in addition to touching every doorknob, he must also quite uncontrollably have to tap his right foot as he touches the knob. The obsession might continue until it becomes quite an elaborate ritual with the individual not only touching the doorknob and tapping his right foot, but perhaps also turning his head three times in alternate directions. It is obvious to see, therefore, how such ritualistic behavior can be psychologically incapacitating and socially inappropriate. With such behavior, the obsessive-compulsive person attempts to alleviate his anxiety. These compulsive acts are repeated in a kind of magical way in order to ward off the engulfing anxiety. They represent routine, which gives the individual a very temporary kind of release from the overwhelming anxiety with which he lives constantly. The obsessive-compulsive is on a psychological seesaw. He is desperately seeking to maintain an emotional balance, only he finds that this balance cannot be maintained. Every compulsive act must be undone by an opposing one. Then, the opposing act must still be reacted to by another opposing act. The individual is in a constant state of fluctuation, doubt, indecision, and ambivalence, not capable of making definite decisions in any direction. His compulsive behavior appears to go on indefinitely.

The compulsions are defense mechanisms in mitigation of anxiety and are frequently symbolic motor rituals which are substitutes for an emotional conflict that the individual has failed to resolve. Obsessive compulsions result from unsuccessful attempts to solve the conflict between a primitive, instinctual drive and the defenses which are raised to control the drive. When the defenses in mitigation of this drive fail, the individual regresses to a previous phase of development and adopts behavior which is reminiscent of one of the earlier stages in growth.

For instance, a child may be obsessed with sexual ideation and engage in compulsive masturbation. The child may even consciously want to stop the masturbation, but may be unable to do so. His masturbation could represent a return to the narcissistic stage of development when all satisfying experiences were autoerotic. This regression, in turn, might be a reaction to the child's original unresolved desire to have sexual relations with a parent (this is a psychoanalytic concept). The child fights this desire, and defends against it by denying the desire and returning to a stage of development where this specific desire was as yet unknown. In this sense, the masturbation is a compulsive act which obscures the original drive, satisfies a related drive, and rids the child of anxiety.

Obsessive compulsions may be either a diagnostic entity in themselves, or a part of other syndromes. It is sometimes difficult to tell when a compulsion neurosis ends and a delusion begins. The compulsion may be so weird or bizarre that it gives the impression of being delusional. The significant difference is the realization by the neurotic that his rituals are irrational, while the psychotic cannot make that distinction. Obsessive-compulsive mechanisms are often a part of the schizophrenic process.

Obsessive compulsions do occur in children, although it is most often not diagnosed as a clear-cut syndrome, but rather as a symptomatic part of a broader clinical picture. Obsessions vary greatly and can range from being simply an ideational wish that misfortune or death befall a parent, to the bizarre, unrealistic persistent thought that one part of the body is growing out of proportion—hands are becoming huge, or the nose is rapidly growing longer, etc. The child knows as well as the adult that the fear is groundless and absurd, but the child fails to understand the significance and symbolism of his compulsions. For instance, the child who must sit in a particular seat, in relation to a particular desk in the classroom, does not understand why he must sit just there. He may even admit the foolishness of such an act, but he feels compelled to do so. If the child is thwarted, great anxiety overtakes him and possible irrationality or aggression toward the thwarting person results. For instance, one such boy, age fifteen, said when he was prevented from sitting in his special chair because another child was occupying the seat, "Well, I guess I'll just have to sit on her face." And he attempted to do just that.

If the compulsion to act is thwarted, the child feels that dire circumstances will result. Compulsions are very frequently seen in connection with phobias. The child who is afraid of attack at night reduces the tension associated with this fear by repeatedly examining the locks on doors, inspecting closets, and looking under beds many times. This compulsive routine gives a sense of security and decreases the obvious fear, although the source of the child's conflict is not the fear itself, but a deeper psychical function which is obscured from consciousness and of which the fear is symbolic.

It is not unusual to find obsessive-compulsive children in the classroom. It is frequently not possible to observe the presence of obsessions unless they are overtly verbally expressed. It is possible, however, to see the many compulsions which children engage in as a defense against the disorganization of the personality by some crippling anxiety. Compulsive children may be excessively orderly and conscientious, always obey instructions to the letter of the law, and be scrupulously methodical in every activity. Their academic work is unfailingly precise, and arithmetic examples are meticulously arranged on the paper, which in turn is creased or folded according to exact measurements. There may be erasures, however, the child having no tolerance for a margin of error, or perhaps no erasures at all because the child uses a new sheet of paper each time there is the slightest error. Their drawings and their other art productions are equally methodical and exact. (See Chapter X, on "The Creative Arts.")

Behaviorally, these children may be excessively punctual, or insist on sitting only in a special seat or standing on line in a special position. They may refuse to respond to a question the first time it is asked, always waiting until the same question is repeated. There are, in fact, an endless variety of ways in which compulsions can operate; the nature of each compulsion is dependent upon the personality of the child involved. There are those children who are compulsive talkers; they never seem to stop talking. When there is a pause in the conversation, they react as if they had to assume the liability of conversation. They talk endlessly, not that they really have something to say; they just seem compelled to keep on talking.

There are also those children who are the "neat children" in the classroom. Frequently the compulsive children, except for the compulsive talkers who may cause many discipline problems in the classroom, are the ones who are praised by teachers for their work and orderliness. In this sense, their compulsions are actually being reinforced by teachers who give them praise. It would be well for educators to recognize that these "model" children, who satisfy the adults' need for orderliness, are not necessarily well adjusted and may be indulging in a rigidity which is symptomatic of maladjustment.

Summary

Neuroses are the result of defenses which have failed to operate successfully. The well-adjusted person uses defense mechanisms successfully. In neurotics, however, there is first a defense against the instinct, then a conflict between the instinctual drive striving for discharge and the defensive controlling forces within the individual. The ensuing conflict raging within the individual causes a repression of the instinctual drive. The final result is the development of a neurotic symptom. The symptom is the only phase of the neurosis which is manifestly observable. Symptoms may be phobias, conversions, or obsessive-compulsive ritual. In neurotics, defensive mechanisms fail to operate and are not serving the individual adequately. The individual feels exposed, unprotected, and helpless in the face of danger, and therefore suffers from a constant overwhelming, extreme anxiety.

Chapter V

Behavior Maladjustments

According to Alexander and Shapiro, the outstanding difference between a behavior maladjustment and a true neurosis is that in maladjusted behavior the unacceptable impulses find outlet in direct action, while in neurosis these impulses are not acted out, but find expression in neurotic symptoms.[1] Behavior disturbance in contrast to neurosis is not merely a private concern of the individual; it also involves the environment. The child acts out his unacceptable impulses in a manner which is often aggressive or antisocial, giving rise to overt conflict with the environment.

Ferenczi has made an analogy between a neurotic symptom and a behavior maladjustment or disturbance.[2] He differentiated between two types of adaptation at the disposal of the organism; first, changes within the organism (for instance, the development of heavy fur on animals in arctic regions), and second, changes in environment (for example, the building of a fire as protection against the cold). Neurotic symptoms exemplify the first category because internal needs are satisfied by an internal process. Behavior disturbances, however, are characterized by the second type, for it is the gratification of needs by activity which directly affects the environment. Such activity, when it

---

[1] F. Alexander and L. B. Shapiro, "Neurosis, Behavior Disorders and Perversions," in *Dynamic Psychiatry,* Alexander & Ross (eds.) (Chicago: University of Chicago Press, 1952), pp. 117–39.

[2] *Ibid.,* p. 132.

is indicative of maladjusted behavior, is unconventional and generally inimical to the best interests of the community. In other words, behavior maladjustment exists when the internal conflict of the child is resolved by the acting-out of conflict in an unacceptable way. For example, a child who is guilt-ridden because of his unconscious death wishes against his father becomes maladjusted if this aggression is turned into bullying, stealing, or any other form of delinquency. On the other hand, another emotionally disturbed child handles the same anxiety attached to the death wish by developing a neurotic symptom, such as a phobia. In the first case, the child becomes a social deviate, and may thereby be considered a behavior problem. In the second case, the child does not antagonize the community—his maladjustment is a source of concern only to his family and himself—but because of the mechanism employed, he may be considered neurotic. Both children, of course, have to be helped. Maladjustments taking the form of severe aggression certainly attain more prominence and are more obvious than neurotic syndromes, which often go undetected. Teachers, however, must be aware of both forms of disturbance and be ready and willing to seek aid for a child. It must be remembered that the difference between a behavior maladjustment and a neurosis can be only the slim line of diagnostic differentiation, just as the difference between normalcy and maladjustment is one of degree rather than kind.

It may be stated succinctly that the normal person may be aggressive if a specific situation calls for aggressive activity; the neurotic person may want to be aggressive, but because of a basic conflict within himself, centered about aggression in relation to passivity, he may develop a paralysis to control the aggression. The behaviorally maladjusted person may become overly aggressive, not only to specific situations, but to all situations, misdirecting his aggression and behaving in an antisocial manner. All maladjustment, it would appear, stems in part, no matter what other factors may be present, from a basic sense of insecurity and a deep feeling of inadequacy and helplessness in the face of overpowering forces which the individual feels he cannot control. The following section will discuss the most prominent types of maladjusted behavior observable in children.

DIRECT OVERT AGGRESSION

Positive Aggression. Aggression is a basic force inherent in man and necessary for human survival. It is a normal characteristic of man, having polemic values, both positive and negative. The true nature of aggression must be clearly determined before it can be labeled in a derogatory fashion.

Aggression has positive values when it involves the kind of self-assertion and domination necessary to the realization of a socially acceptable goal; when the individual, for instance, pursues a course which is beneficial to himself and which is not directed to others in a hostile fashion. This type of aggression gives rise to the educator's search for knowledge, to the proficiency of the doctor in relieving human ills, and to the inventor's drive to alleviate environmental difficulties. Positive aggressive behavior is observed in children who, for example, lead club activities, compete for scholastic honors, or are leaders in their classes. This type of aggression demands that an adult or child must in some measure assert himself and frequently dominate others. In a positive sense, this quality is called leadership. The domination necessary for such leadership is, of course, not socially unacceptable, nor is it offensive to others. For along with the ability to assert himself, the individual also possesses the ability to make others like him and to persuade them to his convictions. Aggression is considered valuable when the motivation behind the particular activity is not only socially acceptable, but frequently individually and socially beneficial. In any social structure, situations often arise which demand a call for social action, imposition of goals upon others, or persuasion of others to perform desired activities. In this sense, leadership qualities are considered positively aggressive.

Negative Aggression. Aggression is evaluated as negative when it takes the form of hostility, expressing itself in a manner which is socially incompatible with acceptable patterns of behavior. This type of aggression gives rise to criminal acts, delinquencies, and other direct defiances of law and order. When aggression takes expression in consistently negative forms it can be defined as a component of maladjustment. Of course, children may be continuously aggressive at home and not exhibit this type of behavior in school, or may consistently be aggressive to very young children and not to peers. Aggression can take many forms and be related to many different situations, but when it is fairly consistent, whether directed inwardly or outwardly, it is an indication of maladjustment.

Overt Aggression. Overt aggression is particularly observable in children who are not as inhibited as adults and who can express their feelings through hostile acts which are antisocial in tenor and in direct defiance of authority and social controls. A lack of inhibition contributes to all types of aggression. This does not mean that children who are uninhibited are necessarily disturbed. But when the degree of uninhibitiveness is extreme, then of necessity social controls are ignored, judgment becomes poor, and the child becomes concerned with self-expression while disregarding societal controls. Aggressive children who indulge in overt aggressive acts, like fighting, bullying, destroying property, or stealing, are labeled by the adult world as "bad," "nasty," or "fresh." Fortunately there are many indications that society is becoming more aware of the fact that overt aggressive behavior is not an expression of mere "badness," but is rather the expression of a disturbed child who is attempting self-preservation.

The aggressive child tries to maintain his status in the world, to achieve some measure of approval, if not from adults then from peers. The need to dominate is constantly present and grows out of a deep-seated feeling of inadequacy along with a basic sense of self-abasement. The aggressive child must constantly prove his own value to the world as well as to himself. Even while personal status is apparently achieved through aggression, the child is really not convinced of his own value and is unhappy in the knowledge that recognition cannot be gained through less violent means. The aggressive child has led a life marked by failure, antisocial activities, rejection, and unhappiness. Approval is sought, but if it is not forthcoming, aggression becomes an attention-getting device which permits the child some means of retaliation for his suffering. It becomes important to the child to be recognized by others, even if not actually accepted, and gratification is obtained from attention, in spite of the fact that it is given in a disapproving manner.

The aggressive child may vocally defy others, fight with little provocation, lie at the slightest opportunity, cheat, steal, truant, debase buildings, destroy property, and in general defy all authority. Any one of these activities, or any combination of them, if this mode of behavior is constant, should be considered an indication of serious maladjustment. The aggressive child, of course, presents a serious discipline problem to the teacher, openly flaunting authority, using obscene language, and destroying both his work and the work of others. Even when the teacher attempts to make a good personal relationship by being especially kind and understanding in response to this unacceptable behavior, the child becomes suspicious and rejects the offer of friendship. He has built up the belief that no adult is to be trusted, and he cannot accept the proffered friendship. The teacher usually heaves a sigh of understandable relief when this type of child is absent from school for any reason, or when chronic truancy becomes his pattern. The teacher realizes that the presence of a disruptive force in class is not only a personal trial, but that other children suffer because of the undue amount of time which must be devoted to this special problem without affording the group any real value from the effort. The overtly aggressive child may not work up to his mental ability, and is frequently a very poor reader. Success is usually foreign to this child, whose pattern has been one of creating disruption, causing chaos, and provoking disciplinary measures which are too often of no avail. The aggressive child is usually not touched by ordinary school punishments, and appears to be immune to shame, embarrassment, or chagrin. School records indicate that these children are labeled by teachers as "troublemakers," "bullies," "obstinate," "fractious," "unruly," and "defiant." Their entire school history may abound with instances of chronic aggressive patterning. The aggressive child is an anxious child who attempts to relieve anxiety and bolster self-esteem by hitting out against the world, which he perceives as hostile. Aggressive conduct can range from mild disobedience to more exaggerated forms of hostile behavior, such as temper tantrums or delinquency. Delinquency stems from the same sources as any other aggressive behavior. It must be considered a symptom of disturbance, developed by a child who is basically maladjusted and who would perhaps, under certain other circumstances, develop neurotic symptoms instead. The delinquent, therefore, has to be considered just as disturbed as a neurotic child. There is no scientific explanation for the "why" involved in the development of a specific type of disturbed behavior. Why, under presumably the same conditions, for instance, does one child become a delinquent; another, a stutterer; a third, a reading disability problem; and a fourth, an obsessive-compulsive? The important factor to be considered is that any one of these symptoms, including delinquent behavior, is indicative of emotional disturbance. Adler [3] states that every child is faced with so many obstacles in life that none ever grows up without striving for some form of significance. Every human being approaches the problem of his personal significance in an individual way. The personality pattern, the development of behavior, and the manifestation of a symptom, whether these expressions appear to be normal or disturbed, are all ways in which children strive for their own significance.

The overtly aggressive child needs to prove his own value through aggressive behavior, which happens to be antisocial in nature and censured by our culture. Such acts as fighting, truancy, thieving, lying, cheating, fire-setting, and cruelty to people or animals, are generally recognized as aggressive. It is necessary, however, to consider the constancy and intensity of the aggressive behavior pattern before it can be considered symptomatic of a disturbance. No one incident of truancy or fighting, no one antisocial act, can be construed as positive evidence of emotional disturbance. One antisocial incident would not be particularly significant, if, for instance, it was precipitated by a particularly traumatic experience which was so overwhelming that the child reacted to it in some temporary form of direct hostile activity. If the antisocial pattern is not constant, the child has managed to resolve the conflict and is able to function again within the structure of society.

In evaluating the degree of severity of a hostile act, it is necessary also to consider whether it is performed in isolation or with a group. A child who is an occasional truant in order to go to a ball game with

---

[3] A. Adler, *Understanding Human Nature* (New York: Greenberg, 1927).

friends, or who engages in occasional thefts because he is a member of a gang and does not want to be considered "chicken," does not present quite as serious a picture as the child who commits thievery or any other antisocial act alone as a result of his own inner promptings. In addition, one symptom alone cannot be evaluated without reference to the entire behavioral picture presented by the child. One form of aggressive behavior usually bears a relationship to other behavior patterns. The child who is a chronic truant, for instance, probably engages in some theft, may lie easily, or shows behavior which may not be aggressive, but which nevertheless is deviate. It must be repeated that constancy of aggressive behavior is an important factor in determining the presence of emotional difficulties. There are some aggressive acts, however, which must be recognized as serious the first time they occur. Even if they are committed but once, they are important indications of maladjustment. A single incident involving such acts as fire-setting, the possession and use of weapons, bodily assault, or sexual perversion are violently aggressive and indicate such poor control and intensity of emotional conflict that their seriousness cannot be minimized.

It is sometimes difficult to evaluate aggressive behavior. The severity of a specific aggressive act is distinguished by the aggressive intent of the child. One must ask whether there is a need for really violent destruction, or whether the act is merely a direct expression of a need for self-assertion. Self-assertive strivings are part of a child's natural development, and unless the intensity of the aggression is such that it reveals strongly destructive impulses, it is merely an attempt to show independence and display power.

Developmental Aggression. Aggressive behavior is one of the ways children have of testing the environment while they attempt to find their independence. Fighting and punching are part of the normal exploratory methods children use in social behavior. The young child who has not yet learned to socialize gives vent to aggressive impulses while struggling with environmental demands. Between the ages of three and nine, fighting in some situations is the natural expression of the child who is learning how to handle frustrations. As the child matures and as concepts of social living develop, control and judgment improve, and there is no longer the need for recourse to direct aggressive activity. A young child is neither rejected by his peers nor by society when he expresses overt aggression. The more he matures, however, the more controlled he is expected to become and the more adult he must behave. The adolescent, therefore, who approaches maturity, learns how to control his emotions on an adult level. In adulthood, the individual is permitted to feel anger, but he is not expected to express this anger in overt aggressive acts. Society places value upon control of the emotions, permitting the adult to show aggression, not in direct acting-out, but rather in verbalization of this aggression.

In a recent study by the authors, it was found that by the time a child reaches adolescence he considers aggressive defiance immature and childish. Even in the choice of a leader, the adolescent, unlike the young child, prefers a new type of person to admire, one who co-operates rather than dominates in leader-group relations. The newly acquired adult manner of self-assertiveness in the older child makes him rebel against the direct aggressive act. When, however, overt aggression as the consistent pattern of response continues past puberty, the adolescent has made little progress toward assuming a realistic adult role and must be considered infantile, immature, and maladjusted.

Robert C.: Male, Age 16, IQ 94

Robert had good school grades, but "D" in conduct from the second grade on. He liked going to school, but he also liked to annoy his teachers. He never played truant because, as he said, "I lived too near the school," but actually he had no desire to be a truant. In school, he would hit other children, call out abusively to the teacher, defy school rules and have temper tantrums whenever the teacher would try to control him. He had few friends because he would antagonize the other children. He was always ready to feel abused by others and to fight them. There often was little provocation for his aggressive behavior, other than, "He looked at me funny," or, "He called my mother a dirty name." He seemed very impulsive, and did not seem to be able to control his aggression. A teacher's estimate of him was "potentially a very dangerous boy who might kill someone some day."

On a psychological examination, it was found that Robert displayed very poor judgment, that he was unpredictable, negative, unco-operative, and very anxious. He had a very poor self-concept and felt inadequate as a human being. He could put no value upon himself as a person and used his hostile impulses as a defense against his basic feelings of worthlessness. He had no control over his hostility, but expressed it directly. He was diagnosed as a primary behavior disorder.

It is evident from the case just presented that Robert was directly acting out his hostility in an attempt to overcome his feelings of inferiority. His aggression was directed against the school; he chose to continue attending school rather than be truant from it. He felt that he could express his aggression against school more readily if he attended than if he were absent. His extreme hostility, however, was not only directed against authority, but against other children as well. It is also interesting to note that Robert was not able to influence others to join him in fighting authority and was rejected by his peers for his excessive aggression. In his particular neighborhood, there were no "gangs" which he could join, and Robert was considered as deviate by the peer group from which he should have received friendship.

Aggressive behavior is an expression of the emotional life of the child. It is a form of communication which reflects the inner storms and tension, giving a glimpse of internal feelings. When a child has to assert himself too violently and too frequently, he has organized his personal social reaction patterns so that his response to society is an angry, aggressive one, frequently destructive and explosively drastic in nature. He has somehow been thwarted in his efforts to maintain some kind of workable emotional balance. By his aggressive behavior he gives evidence of the fight he is putting up against the danger as he sees it of being relegated into oblivion. He has not had the satisfactions of achievement, approval, and security which are essential to growth, maturation and the development of self-respect. This child is not adjusting, and therefore not advancing into maturity. He invades the environment on a brute level, and although he is in dire need of encouragement, direction, and understanding, he fights desperately against receiving them. Because he puts up such a defiant façade, he almost makes it impossible for even those who understand him to like him.

Thus, even those who would offer him the helping hand he so urgently needs, eventually turn away in anger.

COVERT AGGRESSION

There are those forms of aggression which are not usually recognized as aggression because they are not overtly hostile. Hate, jealousy, obstinacy, snobbishness, and righteousness are some forms of aggression which as entities are not considered to be overt. All of these traits, in moderation, are common components of all personalities, and can be defenses used to control and inhibit the direct expression of aggression. These traits are really defenses which are cultivated by mature people to cope with the aggressive impulses they experience but dare not release. The maturing child learns to develop these defenses in an attempt to sublimate overt expressions of aggression. When these defenses break down, however, and when these traits are exaggerated beyond a certain degree, the personality suffers and the child's normal development is threatened.

Jealousy and Hate. Jealousy and hate are subtly related to the expression of anger and fear, and are intimately related to each other in that a child begins to hate as an expression of anger against the person of whom he is jealous or whom he fears. Tendencies to hate appear early in childhood and may achieve a very high intensity in temper tantrums or overt sadism, resolving themselves, perhaps, through milder emotional expressions such as viciousness and nagging. Hate has many directions and can be focused against people and objects, against specific people or racial groups, or against a particular sex or particular objects.

Feeling angry toward the parent and authority is a natural emotion of growing up. The young child is extremely dependent upon his parents. He looks toward them for the fulfillment of his every need. The young baby demands to be fed and changed. The two-year-old insists upon being carried. The five-year-old asks to be read to. Children make constant demands upon their parents without questioning whether they have a right to do so. Essentially they are egocentric, selfish beings who have to learn that gratification cannot be complete. When, therefore, they continue to make demands unrealistically, without awareness of others, and parents do not heed them, they feel angry and hostile toward their parents. The six-year-old who expects the undivided attention of his parents at all times must soon learn that parents have rights also. This lesson can be a bitter one for the young child to accept, and he repeatedly experiences frustration and anger. He may even cry out openly that he hates his mother and father. When the child is disciplined and made fearful of expressing his hate, he does not stop feeling the emotion. Instead, he only stops admitting that he feels it. The child then must suppress the hate, but it does not cease to exist. It may become instead a deep-rooted, heartfelt emotion which seethes within him, giving rise to anxiety and guilt. This is the child who may appear to be "good," but who is nevertheless suffering from deeply felt emotions which he cannot permit himself to express. Because his parents have forbidden him to hate, he feels that the emotion of hating is bad; and, therefore, since he hates, he must be "bad" too. Feelings of inadequacy and self-deprecation, as well as feelings of guilt and anxiety, can then arise. This is the child who becomes a woefully unhappy, maladjusted individual, fearful of his own emotions, haunted by them, and unable to give them expression.

However, the child who expresses his hate does not feel "bad" because of it. He learns that his feelings are not unique although his behavior in reaction to the hate may not necessarily be acceptable. He learns, therefore, to talk over his feelings and relieve his anxiety without resorting to antisocial behavior. The child therefore learns not only to accept his own feelings, but also to control them. In this way the unexpressed hate is not suppressed, to fester inwardly, and to find, perhaps, expression at a later date in an unhealthy pattern or a neurotic outbreak.

During childhood, with growth and maturation, the feelings of hate against parents begin to dissipate, only to rise again in the adolescent years. Although the teen-ager does not really hate his parents, he is struggling against them in his efforts to find his own place in life. During this struggle, his hatred may encompass his teachers, the neighbor next door, and the policeman on the block. Finally, he hates all adults because they represent the authority he not only is struggling against, but with which he also wishes unconsciously to identify. This is the very essence of his difficulty: the desire to be adult while at the same time clinging to the security of his childhood. This then is the basic conflict of adolescence, and should be treated as such. It may appear to adults that the adolescent is angry most of the time, defiant against them, vengeful, and inconsiderate, when actually he may merely be trying out his new independent role. Anything new and desirable has inherent in it an urgency to be exploited to the fullest by most people. Like the adult woman who buys a new hat and creates an opportunity to wear it, so it is with the adolescent who must prove to the world and himself that he is adult. He therefore wears his new-found emotions with blatant, exaggerated pride. He feels everything very intensely, from "adoring" his new teacher, to "loathing" the boy next door, to "despising" his kid sister. Adolescents need a great deal of encouragement at this time to talk over their feelings. The teen-ager who discusses his "pet hate" may soon learn to objectify his feelings by limiting them and directing them against some realistically hateful object, such as a community injustice or a school situation which needs correction.

Jealousy, like hate, is a complex emotion. It is directed not only toward love relationships, but also toward people, their qualities, and property, including siblings, possessions, position, intellectual ability, individual role, or physical appearance. Jealousy is a common trait and most people at some time are capable of experiencing it in moderation and in various relationships.

Jealousy and hate are natural, expected emotional responses, within the experience of all people. If they are all-consuming, however, they may result in distorted attention-getting behavior or excessive dependency. Jealousy in young children is most often evident at the birth of siblings, resulting in regressive infantile behavior, thumb-sucking, soiling, crying, etc. In older children, jealousy and hate may center about scholastic achievement, athletic prowess, or social position. Adolescents are particularly prone to jealousy on a mature level when competing for prominence or striving for success in heterosexual relationships.

When, however, jealousy and hatred give rise to emotions which are so powerful that they precipitate an overt aggressive act, the seriousness of the underlying uncontrolled impulses cannot be overlooked. An all-consuming jealousy can so distort a child's functioning that there is a subsequent distortion of reality, and the resulting behavior is regulated by this distortion. The following case illustrates the devastating result of the lack of detection of the signs of exaggerated hatred and jealousy, serious de-organization of the entire personality.

Tony V.: Male, Age 16, IQ 96

Tony was physically and constitutionally inferior, a child who was hospitalized several times during infancy and childhood. During one of his long hospitalization periods, when Tony was nine, his mother gave birth to a second child. Tony became obsessed with the idea that he was being hospitalized in order to make room for the second child. He was filled with envy and hatred for this child and extended this hate to include all children. He hit other children in the hospital where he was being treated. He directed his aggression particularly against the infants and very young children. He would squeeze, kick, bite and pinch them. After he tried to throw a child out of the window he was removed from the hospital and sent to a psychiatric ward for observation. Upon his return, Tony's relationship to his sibling was an aggressive one, but he attempted to control his aggression with a forced attitude of love, literally "killing the child with love." He would squeeze, pinch and fondle the child with such intensity that the child would invariably cry. While Tony managed to control his aggression at home, he could not, however, do so in the situation outside the home. Tony hit other children in school, again making his particular target the young child. At school, Tony was a severe discipline problem, impulsive in his aggression and defiant of authority. During his school years, he particularly had difficulty with women teachers, being insolent, rude, and defiant. He could not make a good relationship with any woman, whereas he did manage to get along fairly well with men teachers. Five years later, when his mother gave birth to a third child, Tony began to re-experience the same kind of overwhelming jealously that he had experienced with his first brother. This time his maturity gave him a certain degree of insight into the destructive nature of his impulses, and he became so anxiety-ridden and terrified of his own feelings that he admitted himself to a psychiatric hospital, asking to be removed from the environment for fear that he would kill the new child.

It is obvious that hatred and jealousy so permeated this boy's life that the intensity of the emotion grew beyond his means of control. As an adolescent he had still not matured enough to feel that he, himself, could control these impulses, and was forced to ask for assistance from the outside.

Tony's school record during the years between the births of his siblings was characterized by truancy, with abject conformity alternating with violent outbursts of temper. He showed obvious brutality to younger children in the school, and his hatred was clearly so consuming that he distorted reality to the point that all young children became a threat to him. Furthermore, his jealousy of his brothers was directly related to his mother who he felt rejected him in favor of his brothers. His hostility toward his mother found expression in the attitude he developed to all women, as shown in the aggression directed against women teachers.

It is obvious from Tony's history that his whole personality was distorted by his feelings of hate and jealousy. It is also obvious that the pathology that he developed was an attempt on his part to dissipate these feelings, an attempt that proved to be unsatisfactory not only to society, but also to himself.

Righteousness. Adler [4] states that righteousness is an attribute of aggression in that the righteous person is jockeying for a superior position in life by inflicting his morals and standards of living upon others. Righteousness, if not carried to rigid extremes of behavior, can be of benefit to society. Righteousness is not as evident in young children as it may be in adolescence because the young child has not defined for himself the concepts of right and wrong, and is naturally unable to impose upon others moral standards which he himself cannot clearly differentiate. In adolescence, however, ethical values assume greater importance, and the adolescent who is experimenting with concepts of right and wrong readies himself to accept a code of behavior. He attempts to handle the situation not only by accepting the code for himself, but also by imposing this code of ethics upon others. In this way, with the

---

[4] A. Adler, *op. cit.*

imposition of his ethics upon his peers, he tries to reassure himself that his values are reliable.

Imposition of will upon others is a somewhat refined attempt at aggression. It is a defense against the desire to participate in the very activity of which the individual is being critical. This conflict, of course, causes great anxiety. For instance, it is an accepted part of our culture for an adolescent girl to be interested in boys, socialize with them, and attempt to attract them by wearing make-up. The adolescent girl who is critical of her peers because of their interest in boys and who refuses to wear cosmetics on the basis that it is more important to be smart, may be using her intellectualism as a defense against her own instinctual sexual impulses. Righteousness implies not only the imposition of moral standards upon the self and the imposition of will upon others, but also a criticism of others for their lack of acceptance of these standards. Criticism of others is in itself aggressive in nature, and is part of the pattern of righteousness as a defense.

In young children, the individual who is constantly critical of others attempts not only to assume the role of a righteous guardian, but also tries to curry favor in the eyes of adults. This child is the so-called "tattle tale." There is a kind of sadistic component to this type of activity, and when an adult co-operates with the "tattle tale" it reinforces this pattern and encourages its continuance. This behavior permits the child to utilize consistently a defense which results in antagonistic relationships with peer groups.

The righteous child, or the child who carries tales, sets himself apart from the group, attempting to maintain an air of superiority. This child is frequently called a snob, and is frequently in general disfavor with others. The snobbish child may place a high value upon a specific characteristic which he feels he himself possesses to a greater extent than all the rest of the world. He may fixate upon intellectual achievement, social acceptability, personal appearance, etc., all of which can be aggressive in nature. Intellectual aggression is the most subtle of these and is used as an attempt to let others know how superior one's intellect is. Self-esteem, although a part of intellectual aggression, is of no defensive value in and of itself, if the child is not satisfied with his worth, unless others are made acutely aware of it.

This type of behavior, like other defensive patterns, is the result of a basic insecurity which is counterbalanced by an attempt at superiority and an imposition of will upon others. Righteousness, snobbishness, and intellectual aggression are not themselves diagnostic entities, but rather are behavior and personality characteristics which, when carried to an extreme, must be considered components of maladjustive behavior.

Michael I.: Male, Age 15, IQ 140

Although Michael was a good student who made good academic progress, he was considered a difficult child to handle in the classroom. He consistently attempted to correct the teacher, questioning her knowledge and intimidating her by pretending to have a fund of knowledge much superior to hers. At every opportunity he would quote from the classics, paraphrase obscure writers who are not widely read, and mention minute details from historical sources. For example, in an English class, while the group was discussing *Hamlet,* he attempted to show his superiority by incorrectly quoting the metaphysical poetry of the seventeenth-century poet, Abraham Cowley. Frequently, when the teacher investigated the source of his information, Michael's facts were found to be erroneous. When faced with the erroneousness of his information, Michael would seem to be unconcerned, and would counter the criticism with a quote from another equally obscure source. He managed to intimidate not only the teachers, but also the students by his apparent self-assurance and attitude of superiority. He chose his friends carefully, letting them know they were "the chosen few." He maintained a coterie of satellites who called him "the professor" and hung on to his spurious words intently. When Michael decided that school was no longer of value to him, he began to truant, and was admitted subsequently to a psychiatric hospital for observation, after he questioned the authority and judicial knowledge of the judge before whom he appeared on a truancy charge.

It is evident that Michael's difficult interpersonal relationships grew out of his need to impress others with his superiority. His satisfaction came from behavior which was antisocial, distorted, and intellectually aggressive to an exaggerated degree. It is interesting to note that on psychological tests, Michael, who was a comparatively small boy for his age, showed extreme feelings of body inferiority and a great need for approval through intellectual means. Michael's intellectualism seemed to be an overcompensation for his feelings of poor body concept.

Gary W.: Male, Age 9, IQ 105

Gary dogged the teacher's footsteps with stories of, "John wrote on the blackboard," "Cynthia talked," "Juan is chewing gum," etc. He attempted to buy the teacher's favor with tales of misdoings of other children. He consequently had few friends, and when the teacher tried to curb his confidences, he would look forlorn and disbelieving. He never accepted the fact that his stories were not welcome. Although Gary was physically bigger than the other children, he was constantly being beaten by them. He was a very poor fighter despite the fact that he had a good physique, and he could not seem to learn that the aggression against him would stop if he would not carry tales about the other children.

Gary's determination to curry favor is, of course, very evident. He attempted this even when he knew that the other children would hit him. Upon psychological investigation, it became apparent that Gary's problem was centered upon extreme dependency needs. He was constantly looking for a mother figure to love and support him. Because he did not receive such support or approval at home, Gary's behavior became extreme. He sought it from every adult with whom he came in contact. Coupled with Gary's extreme feelings of maternal deprivation was the conviction that he himself was unworthy of being loved. He placed no value upon himself as a human being primarily because he saw himself as an object that his mother could not love. Thus, he rationalized her rejection by accepting the fact that if he were unworthy of love, he must be "bad," and therefore should be punished. Masochistic trends were therefore prominent in his personality make-up. In this way, he accepted the abuse of the other children and even invited it because he believed he should be punished. Thus, his masochistic feelings reinforced his "tell tale" performances.

SELF-AGGRESSION

The aggression considered up to this point has been of the type that is directed outward, hostility which is vented upon the externals in the environment in an attempt to give stature to the individual. A somewhat different type of aggressive behavior, perhaps a more serious problem, because it results in self-destructive activities, is that which is directed upon the self. Self-destructive behavior includes self-inflicted punishment, inciting others to attack (the case of Gary), accidents, and depression. Self-inflicted punishment can be either physical or mental. When it is physical, the child can literally inflict bodily harm upon himself by doing such things as sticking pins in his hands, scratching his skin to the point of bleeding, pulling whole wads of hair from his head, and picking his nose until there is an infection. Nail biting is also a form of self-destruction, but it is rather common and certainly less severe than most other types of masochism.

A child experiences severe mental anguish when he does not wish to preoccupy himself with his difficulties, but still cannot escape from them. Self-torture is based upon self-recrimination, blaming oneself for all adverse conditions of life as they befall the individual, even to the point of assuming blame for events over which the individual clearly has no control. It is the result of a direct expression of guilt feelings from which the individual suffers. All self-aggressive tendencies, whether they be an acute or chronic depression, a specific self-destructive act, or a proclivity for accidents, are the expression of guilt which the child unconsciously experiences and for which he is unconsciously trying to atone. The guilt stems from the fear connected with the uncontrollable instinctual drives which the child feels are base and unacceptable.

Depression. Depression is not difficult to detect because it can be expressed overtly in obvious consistent unhappiness. The child is frequently apathetic, indifferent, and dons a superficial air of boredom. Nothing in life seems to have any value, and he constantly feels unworthy, unacceptable, completely inadequate, and filled with anxiety.

Depressions can lead to psychosis and attempted suicides unless they are recognized as serious and treated promptly. It must be repeated that all maladjustments may lead to serious mental illness, and that the danger signs of disturbed behavior need early detection.

The following case is one example of a depressed adolescent girl who was not given treatment until the depression became so severe that she actually attempted suicide.

Patricia G.: Female, Age 16, IQ 115

Patricia, apparently a "normal" child, came from a fairly good home where her mother was somewhat punitive, but where her father was quite accepting. She had a fairly usual childhood and got along well in school until she entered puberty. At that time, she became apathetic, did not prepare her lessons, sat in class without participating, and seemed to be constantly preoccupied. This behavior continued and became more intense. She began to cry easily, got upset by trivial incidents, and became insensitive about her personal appearance. There seemed to be no way to reach her. Even those with whom she had a good relationship before could not now make any kind of contact with her. This depression resulted in an attempted suicide which culminated in hospitalization.

Depressions at the onset of puberty, when physical and emotional changes take place, are quite common. The difficulty faced in assuming the new role of adolescence is overwhelming to some children. They cannot cope with the additional problems it seems to present and they become anxiety ridden. Suicide is not only an effort to destroy the self, but also an attempt to punish loved ones. In the case presented, Patricia was not only attempting to destroy herself, but was also trying to punish her parents and cause them to suffer. Psychological tests showed that Patricia's conflict centered about the ambivalence she felt toward her mother and the love she experienced for her father. She responded to both of these emotions with overwhelming guilt and anxiety and could resolve this conflict only by an attempt at self-destruction which would serve also to cause her parents anguish. She was trying to retaliate for her misery which she felt they caused by their lack of assistance.

While the teacher does not generally have to face the problem of an attempted suicide in school, there are many manifestations of depression which are discernible in everyday classroom behavior. Depressed children are apathetic, sad, and overly serious-minded. They lack spontaneity and refuse to engage freely and zestfully in any activity. They may answer questions in dull-voiced monosyllables, have few friends, and make few social contacts. They seem not to enjoy things and are unresponsive to fun-provoking situations. They don't seem to get a "kick" out of anything or be able to look with enthusiasm upon any project, even while they might participate and do a good job.

Self-Punishment. A more easily discernible form of self-aggression is overt self-inflicted punishment and obvious provoking of punishment by others. Self-inflicted physical pain expresses itself in such things as hair-pulling, picking at skin, nail-biting, and ear-pulling. It is not infrequent for a child to punch and pull at himself until he is black and blue in spots. The activity amounts to almost a habit which the child doesn't seem to be able to stop. There seems to be no awareness of the actual maltreatment of the body. The masochistic activity apparently relieves the child of anxiety. Under stress situations like a school test, this activity probably will not stand alone as a symptom of maladjustment, but rather will be seen in conjunction with overt aggression and antisocial behavior. The masochistic child often manages to structure his antisocial behavior so that he is caught and punished. Every teacher can recall a child who always seemed to be caught doing something wrong. This is not an accident. The child continues, without being consciously aware of it, to perform in such a way as to be consistently apprehended.

There are also those children who manage to provoke hostile behavior not only from adults, but from peers. They incite aggression against themselves and seem always to be the target for aggression by other children. They are constantly bruised, beaten up, and chronically suffer all kinds of indignities at the hands of their peers. These are the children who tease others, carry tales, direct obscene language at other children, take the belongings of others while they are watching, interrupt play activities, and generally annoy anyone who is around.

This aggression which is turned inward upon the self and is masochistic in nature is also highly pleasurable to these children, frequently indicating some anxiety related to sexual problems. These children derive great pleasure from bodily activities, even bodily abuse, centering their sexual interests upon their own physical bodies, which indicates possible pathological development in sexual areas.

The following case is an example of a child whose aggression was not only directed outward, but who also engaged in masochistic experiences, directing the aggression inward upon herself.

Kathleen F.: Female, Age 7, IQ 72

Kathy was a tubercular baby who was hospitalized for the first two years of life without a mother in the picture. By the time she was seven, she had been tried in four foster homes without success. Her aggressive behavior was impossible to tolerate. At the age of six, she entered kindergarten where, during the first week of school, despite her weak, sickly physical condition, she engaged in unprovoked aggressive behavior by throwing a child down the stairs and crippling him. She was expelled from school and sent for psychiatric observation. Psychiatric investigation revealed that Kathy, because of severe emotional deprivation at infancy, was incapable of making adequate relationships. Kathleen felt that the world was hostile and rejecting, and viewed herself as unworthy of love. After a few months, she was again tried in kindergarten, and a similar aggressive incident caused her to be expelled again. At this time, Kathy began to turn her aggression upon herself by biting her own arms with such force that medical treatment was required. This behavior continued for months and therapy was started. During therapy, Kathy began to make a relationship with the therapist and started to recognize herself as an individual. The biting became less frequent and she again started kindergarten. This time, she was able to control her aggression, both inwardly and outwardly, by adopting compulsive neurotic mechanisms of behavior. She performed all tasks with exactitude, attempting to give herself security, and rigidly maintaining her own prescribed behavioral structure.

Kathleen's aggressive activity was directed both toward the environment and toward herself. According to Bender,[5] children's overaggressiveness is the result of extreme deprivation during the early years. When children are deprived of parental affection, as Kathy was by the enforced hospitalization and the desertion of the mother, they experience the deprivation as an expression of aggression against themselves and counteract this aggression with aggression on their own part. The child feels there can be no worse deprivation than the one already suffered and counteracts this deprivation with aggressive be-

---

[5] L. Bender, "Genesis of Hostility in Children," *American Journal of Psychiatry,* 105 (1948), 241–45.

havior. Aggression can, of course, also be an attention-getting mechanism, and be used as a substitute for affection. The masochistic components of this type of personality patterning are the result of a feeling of utter and desperate worthlessness, based upon unconscious reasoning that if one does not have the love needed, one is not worthy of love; and the blame for not getting this love is turned inward upon the self. Spitz has done some studies in deprivation of love in infancy [6] and indicates that there are evidences of depression and self-inflicted pain, even to the point of death, in infant behavior as well as in that of older children. Ribble has also drawn the same conclusion in her studies.[7]

A less obvious form of masochistic behavior is seen in children who are accident prone; they too turn their aggression inward upon themselves. The child who seems to be constantly in accidents is trying to inflict pain and punishment on himself because of his own feelings of unworthiness. Having an accident is also his way of controlling the overt aggression with which he might abuse the world. Aggressive behavior, regardless of the form of expression, is based on general feelings of anxiety, the desire for power, and possessiveness. The child who does not get what he wants construes this as deprivation on the part of the parent. Aggression is, therefore, directed not only at the environment in general, but also at the parent who is the controlling force. The child then hates the parent, has hostile aggressive wishes which are directed against the parent, and experiences guilt because of these wishes. In order to alleviate the guilt feelings and control the aggressive impulses, he turns the hostility upon himself. The ultimate in self-aggression results in suicide or suicidal wishes. Death, of which the child has no real concept, is a solution to an overwhelming problem, and at the same time causes suffering to the adults in the family constellation. Death has no finality in the child's thinking. The child conceives of a recovery from death in the same way that he views the toy soldiers whom he kills and then resurrects in play situations. In this way, running away from home can be part of the same pattern.

---

[6] R. Spitz, "Anaclitic Depression," *Psychoanalytic Study of The Child* (New York: International Universities Press), II (1946), 313–42.

[7] M. Ribble, *The Rights of Infants* (New York: Columbia University Press, 1943).

The child views running away as a punishment directed toward the parental figure, but also directed against the self. The child's running away is a punitive experience as well as a wished-for one. The child runs away to punish his parents. At the same time, feelings of worthlessness overcome him, because he wouldn't be running away in the first place unless he felt unloved and rejected by the parent. Running away is usually immediately preceded by an incident in which the child is chastised by the parent for some reason. The chastisement is interpreted by the child to mean rejection and the child feels unloved and unwanted as well as aggressive and rebellious. Feelings of unworthiness develop in the child and result in feelings that "if they don't love me, I must be bad." The running away then represents aggression both to the parents and to the self, a retaliation to the parent as well as a self-punishing experience.

A group of disturbed children, patients at a psychiatric hospital, were asked how they could best retaliate against parents when they were most angry with them. The following are representative answers of several age groups:

CHARLES, Age 10: "If my father hated me, I'd kill myself."

SEON D., Age 7: "Kill myself if I wanted to get even. If they don't care for me, I don't care for them. No, maybe I'd kill my mother 'cause I wouldn't be worth a plug nickel if I were dead."

NESTOR, Age 11: "Just run away, the worst thing I could do, man. You make your mother feel sorry and bad. She has to look for you all night. Some guy might come and take you away forever, and you might be hurt for good sometimes."

WALTER, Age 10: "I'd run away to midnight, get into trouble and have a lot of fun."

WALTER, Age 9: "Run away, I guess. I'd scare my mother."

DENNIS, Age 6: "I would take a nap."

CHARLES, Age 14: "I'd run away, and they'd be sorry, maybe even to Philadelphia."

MIRIAM, Age 15: "I wouldn't eat. She'd get worried."

It is evident from these answers that aggression is not only directed in every case toward the parent, but that aggression was also turned upon the self. Some children thought of openly killing themselves, while others suggested using withdrawal as a means of aggression. They suggested taking a nap, or simply not eating; in this way they would punish the parent as well as themselves. Children may also equate going to bed with punishment. The greatest number of children, however, simply wanted to run away. It is interesting to note that in one case, the running away was fraught with danger, for the child believed he might be taken away by a stranger and hurt. In this case, the thought of self-punishment was exceptionally strong and may have had sexual components. In the same way, accident proneness is also an aggressive act which is subjected upon the self and punishes the loved ones. The child who always seems to have accidents is not merely unlucky, but is seeking opportunities to atone for guilt and feelings of unworthiness. Although there are such phenomena as true accidents, the child who always seems to be in the way of a car, or who frequently falls downstairs, or who gets hit by balls, etc., is unconsciously punishing himself for the unconscious conflicts he experiences, whatever they may be, as well as attempting to reassure himself that his injuries are of concern to his parents.

Summary. Aggression is an innate instinctual impulse which may give rise to a need for aggressive behavior. Aggression which can be successfully sublimated may become socially useful, while overt aggression which is destructive in nature is an acting-out of the child's need to inflict pain and punishment upon himself or upon others. Aggressive behavior which is uncontrolled is an easily observed, obvious indicator of maladjusted behavior.

WITHDRAWAL MECHANISMS

The denial of unpleasant reality is a normal phase of development. Young children refuse to recognize that which is painful to them. They invent fathers, for instance, when the father is dead; they phantasize a new reality in which they have a father. Denial, however, is used as a defense by the very young, and ceases to be effective when the child becomes five or six. If denial, as a mechanism, continues into later years, it is a regression to a previous level and represents immature behavior.

Withdrawn children frequently use their phantasy as part of the mechanism of denial. They substitute phantasy for reality. Participating in everyday activities can be a painful experience to the withdrawn child, who is concerned with phantasy and who has little or no ability to engage in social intercourse. The child who establishes a behavior pattern of refusal may do so not only to protect himself against failure, but also to retaliate for whatever intolerable pressure is being exerted upon him. Withdrawn children are often overcompliant, passive, or apathetic. Maladjustments of this type are difficult for adults to detect because, being without any overt aggressive elements, the withdrawn child is generally looked upon with favor. He is not a troublemaker, is seen and not heard, is rarely rambunctious or rude, and generally does what he is told. He may be regarded as sweet, quiet, or even painfully shy, as "no trouble at all."

Phantasy. Some withdrawn children seem to have inner resources which compensate for a lack of friends and a lack of social ability and gregariousness. They enjoy isolated activities and seem to be literally "lone wolves," seeking companionship from no one. Despite outward appearances of pleasant apathy, the withdrawn child is basically an unhappy child who leads an active inner life to compensate for personality deficiencies. The withdrawn child wants desperately to be successful in his interpersonal relationships, to have friends, to be well liked, and to be independent. Withdrawn behavior is rooted in passivity and compliance, because the child uses these to seek approval from others, fearing that if passivity is not maintained, rejection by others will be the result. In order to compensate for this passive outward existence, in which all aggressive impulses are stifled, a rich inner phantasy life is developed. In this life the child assumes all the characteristics which he does not actually possess, but which he desires. Phantasy, or daydreaming, is an escape to a dream where actions are completed, energies are spent, aggression is expressed, and the child's self-esteem is heightened. Even daydreams in which the child is beset by extreme difficulties and horrible accidents of fate can be considered mechanisms of fostering self-esteem, as the child invariably phantasies himself as overcoming and conquering extreme catastrophe. The child may develop the ability to withdraw mentally from any group in which he finds himself, and become preoccupied with phantasy. At such times, when phantasy is so intense, the child may not even hear when he is spoken to. He generally has an extreme need for acceptance, however, and when he appears to be rude and indifferent at such times, it is because of this preoccupation with a rich world of phantasy which he utilizes to compensate for those personality characteristics that he wants, but does not actually possess. The withdrawn child needs so much emotional support that at times he literally clings bodily to an adult in seeking this physical support. Young children, especially, cling to parents when they need reassurance. By the time a child reaches school age, however, this clinging should no longer continue; the child should have developed more independent attitudes. When bodily clinging continues in school, the withdrawn child may be adding another symptom of immature behavior to his inadequate basic patterning.

This need for acceptance makes the withdrawn child easily susceptible to any form of criticism, which causes painful emotional experiences for him. This vulnerability can result in a great deal of crying and in oversensitivity to the difficulties of everyday living. The withdrawn child sees himself as unloved and unacceptable, and develops the withdrawn pattern of response to allay his feelings of discomfort and pain. These very patterns, however, are so self-defeating that they preserve the very attributes which are responsible for this negative self-concept.

Phantasy, of course, is one of the normal components of everyone's inner mental life. All people phantasize, whether it be to future periods of prosperity or to particular situations of self-aggrandizement. Phantasy is normal, and certainly, in children, it is particularly to be desired. It is the mechanism through which children meet and overcome failures and satisfy themselves in periods of particular stress and frustration. Phantasy, in normal children, however, takes second place to realistic socialization and friendships. Normal children generally relegate their phantasy to privacy, always preferring direct socialization to their phantasy. It is only when phantasy is extremely bizarre, without the child's recognizing its bizarreness, or when it is so pervasive that the child relinquishes his contact with the environment to a large degree in order to continue phantasizing, that phantasy is unhealthy.

Phantasy can often be communicated to others by written composition. The following composition was written by a child, age twelve, who was asked to write about "My Favorite Daydream."

"I went to Mars with my father, but first my father had to get a rocket. He got the rocket and off we went to the moon and Mars. First, we stopped at Mars. That was fun, except those little strange men fought us and almost killed us, but we got away. When we got away, we got to the moon. There were other men there, even worse than on Mars, but they don't fight us because we got the spray gun which we captured from the men on Mars. So we got away safe and brought back a million dollars which a scientist who got there first, but who had died there, had left."

The boy who wrote the story was an extremely shy, withdrawn child, who rarely volunteered in class and who did not have many friends. He would stammer when called upon and usually did not know the lesson for the day. It is apparent from this composition that this boy had an active phantasy life and compensated in phantasy for the aggression he did not display in real situations.

When phantasy is bizarre, it may reach the proportions of hallucinations and delusional systems, culminating in a full-blown psychosis. When phantasy is all-pervasive, the child continues to retreat from socialization, making the phantasy more important than reality. In these cases, when phantasy is accompanied by withdrawal, it must be considered symptomatic of serious mental illness.

Lack of Phantasy. The blotting out and blocking of meaningful content is apparent in children even when there seems to be a superficial social adequacy. Withdrawal can be manifested in a lack of emotionality and a fear of emotional involvement. Children can be withdrawn and anxious, inhibiting the interplay between themselves and the environment on an emotional level, while their overt behavior appears socially acceptable. They attempt to maintain a defense against the overt violation of reality while paying a price for this maintained reality in the form of self-restrictions on an emotional level. They overcontrol their emotions, repressing overwhelming emotionality and abandoning the usual interpersonal involvements. The lack of emotional investment in relationships is difficult to observe in the usual, casual daily contacts. These children are sometimes so inhibited in emotional affect that their inner phantasy is blocked and their fear of expressing themselves is evident in academic areas, particularly in the language area. They sometimes present an incongruous picture of high intellectual ability with poor functioning in imaginative expression. They are so fearful of revealing themselves that they do poorly in activities which require phantasy, like oral and written composition. They seem devoid of any resources on this level, and although their abilities are apparent in many factual areas, they cannot draw upon themselves for stimulation and satisfaction involving reflection and achievement by means of creative productions.

The following composition was written by such a child, age nine, who was asked to write a composition about any topic he chose. He wrote:

"James came to school in a bus. Betty came to school in her new little shoes. Jimmy came to school on a blue bicycle. Jack came to school in his uncle's car. Mary came to school."

This composition was based upon the child's reader and in no way divulged any emotional content. This child, who was of superior intelligence, could not permit himself any phantasy. He was completely blocked emotionally, and if one were to judge his capacities from those written and verbal productions which did not depend upon learned facts, the picture presented would be completely false.

Summary. The pattern of withdrawal can be based upon goals which are beyond the scope and achievement of a child. Rather than face the knowledge of his own inadequacies and probable subsequent failure, the child refuses to recognize his own goals and inner demands, turning away from facing himself as well as from facing society. Such a child is usually considered to be shy, well mannered, and easily disciplined. The withdrawn child may blush readily, become embarrassed easily, and be overly sensitive. In former periods of culture and education, the child who was "seen, but not heard" was considered to be the model child. Today, it is recognized that such behavior is really a form of maladjustment which, when chronic, can lead to serious mental illness.

SUMMARY

Maladjustments are defined in this chapter by the recognition of expressed deviate traits in the development of defensive behavior. All people utilize defensive behavior and perform certain acts designed to eliminate both internal and external dangers. These self-preservative acts may be either defensive or offensive and relate to conflicts in either flight or fight patterns. When the flight pattern predominates, the result is withdrawal, and when the fight pattern is dominant, the behavior becomes aggressive. Both aggression and withdrawal are normal components of every personality if these characteristics are balanced in such a way that the resultant behavior is both acceptable to society and satisfying to the individual. When the withdrawal or aggression, however, takes on exaggerated modes of expression, invades the environment with its unacceptability, and imposes limitations upon the individual's capacity for both work and enjoyment, it is indicative of the unresolved, unconscious conflict with which the individual is struggling, and serves as a warning that the instinctual impulses and the guilt associated with them are too difficult for the individual to resolve.

Chapter VI

Sexual Deviations in Children

The mores of our culture prescribe the acceptable sex practices to which both children and adults are expected to conform. Various cultures, at different times in history, as well as in the present, and in various parts of the world, have well-developed, rigid codes of sexual behavior giving testimony to the unexpressed, but clearly understood concept of the intensity of the sexual drive in the human being.

As discussed previously, the sexual instinct is a strong, innate drive which has to be controlled by the individual. The course of the development of this control begins in early childhood. The child learns that in the society of which he is a member, certain types of behavior are taboo.

Normal Sexual Development

Infancy. The infant is not able to differentiate between the physical self and the world. The distinction between crib or mother and the self is not clearly defined in infancy. Infant behavior functions in terms of gross level responses to basic body needs, with emotional reactions intertwined in the gratification of these body needs. There is a complete unawareness of the environment. The infant is completely helpless, functioning on an instinctual level as a dependent, demanding organism.

As the infant matures, perceptions become enlarged to include not only the various persons and objects which are familiar to him, but also his own physical body. The infant begins to explore his body, trying to suck his hands, examining his toes, trying in this way to define and separate the concept of self from the environment. He also begins to recognize his mother and to react to affection. This period of body exploration—touching and stroking himself—not only clarifies for him the limits of his body, but also gives him pleasure. He is narcissistic in the sense that he views himself as the center of the world, with the people who inhabit his world existing only to serve him. His needs are merely the sensuous ones related to feeding, caressing, and elimination.

Beginnings of Maturation. By the time the child is one year old, he is faced with the knowledge that he is expected to conform to certain demands put upon him by his parents, namely, in the area of elimination. Toilet training is experienced by the child as an invasion of his autonomy. The rapidity with which a child is toilet trained elicits from most parents feelings of either displeasure or pleasure. When the child is amenable to toilet training, the parent may shower the child with approval, and this approval is interpreted by the child to mean that he is loved. Conversely, the child who for various reasons, either physiological or psychological, is delayed in his training and faces the subsequent disapproval of the family, interprets the disapproval as rejection and denial of love.

The child then interprets the toilet-training process as an affectional relationship between the self and parents, and he discovers that this first act of free will (willingness to control elimination mechanisms) may be used as a weapon against the parents. When the goal is to displease the parent, the child soils; when the aim is to gain affection and approval, there is conformity. The child who conforms to these first parental demands may become the child who adapts easily to other persons and to societal controls, which are the natural extensions of parental controls. On the other hand, the child who defies the parents may extend this defiance with behavior directed against other controls imposed upon him.

This period of toilet training is particularly significant in the sexual and emotional development of the child. For the first time in the child's life, activities are governed by an ability to control elimination functions. Some parents emphasize the importance of this control by constantly asking the child if there is a need for elimination. Trips cannot be taken and visits cannot be made unless the child is first seated on the toilet. Toilet training can be the directing force of a child's life during this period. Not only is the child aware of the importance of the eliminative process, but he also, in handling the genitals, develops an acute awareness of sexual organs and of the secondary pleasure experienced in manipulating them.

The child invests the sexual organs with the same values parents place upon the process of elimination. The parent who places undue stress upon the sexual organs and their role in elimination processes, may cause the child great anxiety relating to genitalia, even after toilet training is accomplished. Psychoanalysis has indicated that adult sexual behavior is frequently related, at least in part, to the parental attitudes the child experienced in relationship to toilet training.

The frequent manipulation of the genital area is a source of pleasure to children and often results in masturbatory activity. Again, parental attitudes become of paramount importance. The child who is taught that genital organs are "dirty" and "nasty" and who is punished for occasional masturbation, may begin to believe that all activity associated with genitalia is offensive. Thus, natural processes of growth and development begin to be viewed with anxiety and guilt, whether there is actual open masturbation or merely the desire for it.

The child of two or three is aware of his sexual organs, likes to play with them in a pleasurable fashion, and may begin to be exhibitionistic. This exposure, dependent upon the personality of the child, may be the result of the child's need to flaunt authority, or a need to determine the limits of acceptable behavior, or a resentment toward the confinement of clothing. Stated in another way, the boy who has been permitted full freedom of sexual expression, and is unaware of prohibitions, may take out his penis in front of his mother's guests in an effort to determine just how far he must go to obtain restrictions from authority. The same motivation may prompt a girl to lift up her dress and ask to be admired. These children are trying to set the limits of social behavior and to determine for themselves a code of behavior by which they can abide. Another child with the same behavior may be defying parents with an aggressive sexual act which he consciously recognizes as being wrong. A third child may be just experimenting with body parts without any awareness of a need for limits, or any knowledge of the rightness or wrongness involved.

A child of three or four engages not only in body exploration of his own, but in exploration of the bodies of other children. Children are very curious about the opposite sex, and if their natural tendency to explore the body of another child has been limited, they will enter into play activities which can resolve their curiosity. Such children "play doctor" and use this experience to satisfy their own curiosity. Parents quite often forbid boys and girls to explore each other's bodies, and also forbid children of the same sex to manipulate each other's bodies. Children, therefore, must resort to any play situation which will satisfy their own needs and which, at the same time, will not conflict with their parents' code of acceptable behavior.

Sexual Identification. Children at the age of three or four who become conscious of their own bodies and curious about the opposite sex, also at this time begin to identify with the parent of the same sex. Little girls are encouraged to play with dolls, play house, and, in general, to be the mother in play activities. They attempt to imitate the parent of their own sex, to accept both the interests and the behavior which relate to this parent, and in general, identify with the parental role. Similarly, little boys are given guns and airplanes to play with and are expected to participate in the more aggressive games because traditionally the masculine role in our society tends toward accentuating the assertive aggressive components of human behavior. Boys, then, begin to identify with the father, while girls begin to identify with the mother.

This process, whereby children accept the role of their own sex by aligning themselves with the parent of the same sex, is known as identification, and by the time a child is four or five, this identification should be fairly well set. Difficulties in adequate identification can lead to many types of pathologies in personality development. The child of seven is already fairly well identified with his own sex, not only with the parental figure, but with peers. Children during this period develop strong, close friendships with children of their own sex and even may deride children of the opposite sex. This period lasts until the onset of adolescence, and is the time of peer group activities, clubs devoted exclusively to one sex, and interests outside the realm of heterosexual activities.

Adolescence. Interest in the opposite sex becomes reawakened at adolescence, when boy-girl relationships become a prime factor in preparation for adulthood. This is the period for the development of secondary sex characteristics, and the adolescent is once again aware of himself physically and overly concerned with body sensations, but this time primarily in terms of heterosexuality. The adolescent period is characteristically one of great psychological stress during which attempts are made to assert independence, to accept the adult sexual role, and to conform to societal pressures regarding acceptable sexual behavior.

The adolescent who is developing concepts of how a person should behave, struggles with many impulses at the same time while attempting to exert control over them. There is a conflict between satisfying needs and conforming to morality and the dictates of conscience. Adults, in general, are not aware of the intensity of the adolescent struggle and tend to treat it with condescension and amusement. This attitude merely adds to the difficulty. Physically and biologically the adolescent is ready for the adult sex role, while socially, economically, and emotionally, adult maturity is not yet attained. This hiatus between the two extremes has to be accepted, integrated, and leveled off, adding to the sense of frustration and inadequacy that is part of normal adolescent development.

RELATIONSHIP OF SEX DEVIATIONS TO MALADJUSTMENT

Sex deviations are indicative of maladjustment and may occur as part of a larger picture of malfunction. Sexual abnormality may be part of a psychosis or neurosis, or be evidence of a conduct disorder. No particular sex deviations are significant of a specific disease entity, nor are they relegated to particular age levels. They may occur in early childhood as well as in adolescence. It must be emphasized, however, that a particular act cannot be labeled as deviate without consideration being given to the normal behavior of a particular age level. For example, when a four-year-old child exposes himself it hardly has the significance it would have were the child fifteen. It is not enough to classify sexual deviations as behavior patterns in and of themselves. Sex deviations can be a part of many types of maladjustment, and under most conditions should be considered as merely one indication of a pathology.

Excessive Masturbation. Masturbation is one of the commonest forms of sexual gratification and is the most accessible way to meet unrequited sex impulses for either sex at any age level. Masturbatory activities as such cannot be considered a sexual deviation unless they are indulged in excessively. Inappropriateness, again, has to be considered from the point of view of both age and place. Certainly a three- or four-year-old may masturbate openly without being aware of the fact that the act is socially offensive. However, as the child matures, he accepts the censure of adults, and when the impulses become too strong for control, masturbation may occur but only in privacy. The young child has not yet learned what is socially acceptable, and is not giving evidence of maladjustment when masturbation is practiced in public. But an eleven-year-old who could not maintain control and masturbated in public would most likely be showing signs of some kind of emotional disturbance. The very young child, generally, masturbates out of a need to gratify a simple physical body pleasure. There is no heterosexual connotation to the activity and no orgasm. Between the ages of seven and eleven, there is comparatively little open masturbation under normal conditions, because the infancy period of body exploration is ended and the child turns his attention to other activities. The adolescent, however, is sexually stimulated in an adult sense, so that adolescent masturbatory practices are accompanied by phantasy relating to the opposite sex. They usually culminate in an orgasm.

When a child is disturbed, masturbation may be excessive, occurring most frequently at times of particular stress regardless of the social setting. At school age, masturbation in a classroom or in any social group setting is *always* an indication of disturbance because it is inappropriate. By the time a child is six, there should be control over instinctual sexual drives so that masturbation in public should not occur. In a school situation, when the drive is so strong and control so poor that there is overt masturbation, it becomes apparent that the child is anxiety ridden. The act of masturbation is used as a means of releasing tension by resorting to infantile behavior. In this sense, masturbation is a regression to an earlier period of development and is an immature effort to resolve an anxiety problem.

Masturbation can, under certain conditions—particularly when other grossly deviate behavior is in evidence—be just as bizarre as any other manifestation of serious illness. A group of disturbed children were observed over a period of three months in a special class, and isolated instances of masturbatory activities were noted. The bizarre quality of the masturbation was evident on many different occasions. An adolescent boy was seen masturbating with a typewriter ribbon. A rather young girl held her vagina almost throughout the day. A small group of boys about ten or eleven years old listened to a song on the radio which repeated the refrain, "Please don't squeeze the banana," and masturbated openly each time it occurred. These instances, of course, are extremely bizarre, and occurred under the special conditions of a school in a psychiatric hospital, where there was no censure of this behavior. The teacher of the regular classes can be alerted to evidences of masturbation and should recognize that such behavior is symptomatic of maladjustment and not an expression of a "dirty" mind.

Exhibitionism. Most children learn at an early age to control their exhibitionistic tendencies. Certainly by the time a child is old enough to enter school these impulses should be successfully repressed. Children who explore their genitals may do so out of a need to gain attention in a sexually aggressive manner. They may also be showing an exaggerated sexual concern, choosing to disregard controls of which they are aware. These children are overly anxious about sexual activities, and this concern may occupy their conscious thoughts in a compulsive manner. While a child may recognize the moral turpitude of a sexual act, he may nevertheless not be able to control it. Exhibitionism, particularly in the older child, is a form of sexual stimulation which represents a deviation in sexual development and which may become a substitute for normal sexual activity. It is a form of sexual behavior which is aggressive and which is intended to shock members of the opposite sex. In this sense it is a sadistic activity, which when indulged in by boys, for example, is directed toward making a girl suffer, deprecating her femininity. Such boys have poor interpersonal relationships with women. This is attributed in psychoanalytic theory to an unhealthy attitude toward the mother figure.

Eugene H.: Age 14, IQ 111

Eugene was ungovernable and delinquent at home as well as in school. He was expelled from school because of destructive assaultive behavior which disrupted the whole class. In school, as well as at home, he was sadistic and threatening to others. He was admitted to a hospital after an episode of exhibitionism when he exposed his genitals in public. Psychological investigation revealed that Eugene was preoccupied with aggressive drives toward his peers and was frustrated in interpersonal relationships. He was asocial and had only the most derogatory attitudes toward people, which grew out of his inability to make genuine human identification. He was very critical of himself and had very strong feelings of inadequacy. He wanted to be virile and manly, but felt himself inadequate. He could not accept women, feeling they were hostile and rejecting and "good for sex only."

DIAGNOSIS: Primary behavior disorder with neurotic traits.

It is evident from Eugene's history that his aggressive behavior was overcompensation for his feelings of worthlessness. He used aggressive behavior to attempt to prove his own masculinity to himself. His feelings of unworthiness, coupled with his critical and hostile attitude toward women, resulted in behavior which was not only aggressive to peers, but also sexually assaultive to women. Boys who are sexually assaultive to women frequently are not assaultive because of sexual stimulation alone, but because they suffer from a deeper pathological process.

Girls, on the other hand, even when disturbed or concerned with sexual matters to an intensified degree, usually do not resort to overt exhibitionistic acts because our culture encourages them to dress, walk, and talk in a sexually provocative manner. These girls can take advantage of our social structure to mold their exhibitionistic tendencies within the framework of accepted heterosexual behavior. However, there are those girls who obviously overexpose themselves and seem to invite sexual assault. These girls may be really disturbed and unable to control their exhibitionistic impulses.

Sex Play. In the normal course of development a certain amount of so-called sex play is expected exploratory behavior. As mentioned earlier in this chapter, young children may "play doctor" and engage in some type of physical contact with each other in games like tag, wrestling, tug of war, leapfrog, etc. Physical contact is an inherent quality of these games and children derive pleasure from the contact, whether it is related to members of the same sex or the opposite sex. It is not uncommon to see seven-year-old children, for example, roll over each other on the floor, looking as if they were in mortal combat. When separated by concerned adults they look up, surprised, and say, "He's my friend."

Older children and adolescents engage in normal sex play which is heterosexual and which is an attempt to make adult relationships. At social gatherings such games as "spin the bottle" and "post office" are accepted as normal evidences of maturation.

Sex play as it is exhibited by disturbed children, however, is somewhat bizarre, exaggerated in importance, and inappropriate to a situation. Disturbed children may be interested in animal sex behavior in an inappropriate way, stopping to ask the sex of an animal in a story, or insisting that a specific sex be given to specific animals in a fairy tale. *The Three Little Pigs* may become two man pigs and a girl, to one child; another child may ask for the sex of an elephant in a specific story where there is no connotation in the story itself suggesting the sex of the animal.

Children may give evidence of a perverted type of sex play by directing their attention to the examination of animal genitalia, even to the point of sexually stimulating an animal or attempting sexual intercourse with an animal. This distorted expression of the sex drive may manifest itself in direct, cruel, sadistic behavior upon the animal. Sadism, whether directed upon animals or upon other children, has sexual features even when it is not directly or overtly sexual in nature. Sadistic acts may range from mild teasing to the most extreme brutality.

Subtly related to sadism is masochism, which is the turning of sadistic impulses inward upon the self. Masochism may be another manifestation of perverted sex play, ranging from minor things like excessive nail-biting and skin-pinching to the serious and dangerous inflicting of severe pain upon the self or the inducing of others to do so.

Perverted sex play is occasionally seen in young children who are so severely disturbed that they may attempt to have intercourse with other children and adults. Such children are precocious in their sexual drives and exhibit what could be considered adult provocative behavior. They may appear to be trying to establish coy, teasing, mature heterosexual relationships incongruous to their age, or they may simply manifest an unhealthy, uninhibited interest in sexual matters.

Precocious sexual behavior is completely inappropriate in the young immature child, and usually indicates a serious disturbance. On the other hand adolescents who are just entering adulthood may indulge in teasing, coyness, and seductive behavior, and this behavior is normal for the stage of growth and development at this age. However, when these sexual concerns assume undue proportions and exclude all other interests, a disturbance is clearly evident.

Sexual preoccupation, whether it be in young children or in adolescents, can indicate an unhealthy mental state. Such preoccupation implies the complete absorption of the child in sexual matters, destroying the motivation to participate in other activities. For example, a young child uninhibitedly asked, "Teacher, how many children you got?" When he received the answer, "Three," he said, "Well, she must have done it at least three times." Such concern, evidence of sexual preoccupation, entered every phase of his school work. When he worked in clay, he "made penises"; he drew pictures of "naked girls" in drawing class; and when he wrote a story, he chose the topic, "When I Get Married." Even arithmetic did not escape; his arithmetic notebook was full of insinuations like "woman divided by man gives baby," and he called it division.

The manifestations of this child's overwhelming preoccupation with sex would represent a disturbed pattern at any age level for any child. Only a disturbed child could so freely indulge in this type of behavior so consistently and with such a lack of inhibition.

Obscenities. Obscenities represent one of the most difficult classroom problems. It is the most frequently encountered form of sexual concern, utilizing a verbal or written insinuation which is aggressive in nature, and not infrequently directed toward the teacher. It is often difficult for the teacher to view obscenities objectively, and the important fact that flagrant use of obscene language can be an expression of maladjustment is too easily disregarded. Obscenities may be regularly used as part of everyday speech patterns, particularly in the more deprived areas of large cities; children from these areas naturally would not attach great importance to their use in conversation. When, however, obscenities are loudly directed toward the teacher or used excessively in a formal classroom situation, it must be considered as evidence of deviant behavior. Ferenczi states that all obscenities stem from aggression which is sexual in nature.[1] It is the direct outpouring of a primitive sexual impulse. Those obscenities which imply sexual perversion or incestual relationships generally provoke the strongest response. The child who is merely angry may say, "F—— you." In a rage he increases his obscenity to, "You are a mother f——." Or, in a personal attack, he insinuates a perversion by calling another child a "faggot." Children who are more adept at controlling the impulse to use obscenities, but who nevertheless feel the need for this type of aggression may cloak it, for example, in such intellectualisms as "Father, uncle, cousin, kin— use first letters only," or they may attempt to veil the sexual content by an inferred aggression like, "Your father tests toilet paper—and not with his nose."

When obscenities are used in peer groups their significance is somewhat less than when they are expressed in the presence of authority figures. When directed against authority it represents not only defiance, but a lack of adequate control, and poor judgment.

The child who cannot verbalize his obscenities may express them by

---

[1] S. Ferenczi, *Sex in Psychoanalysis* (New York: Basic Books, 1950), pp. 132–53.

resorting to pictorialization. Some children may express obscene thoughts in surreptitious doodlings, while others, more defiant, may draw pictures clearly related to heterosexual sexual relationships and flaunt them in the teacher's face. Such pictures are frequently passed about the room, causing commotion, and literally forcing the teacher to take some sort of action. These drawings are similar in nature to verbalized obscenities and indicate an excessive concern with sexuality.

Homosexuality. Perhaps the severest form of sexual deviation, the least amenable to change and the most significant in the entire life pattern of a child, is homosexuality. Homosexuality is an abnormal developmental process which appears to stem from a distortion in sexual identification. Boys, who should identify with the male role, and girls, who should identify with the female role, somehow fail to do so completely. Because they fail to make an adequate identification with their own sex, their relationships to the opposite sex must of necessity also be disturbed. Thus, in a homosexual relationship, even though a male may take the masculine role or a girl may take the feminine role, the disturbance still exists, because they are able to play their roles only with members of the same sex. Generally, however, this group may be considered less "sick" than those homosexuals who play the opposite role, that is, men who play the female part and women who play the male role. There are various schools of thought concerning the causes of homosexuality. The psychoanalytic schools attribute this type of malfunction to a regression to a period in childhood when the child fails to make an appropriate identification with the parent of the same sex. Other theories consider homosexuality to be the result of an endocrine disbalance or a biological deficit. In the normal process of sexual development, both feminine and masculine traits are expressed, worked out, and resolved. For example, the masculine child, although he may have certain feminine components, is able to make an adequate identification with the masculine role, and the male components become dominant in his personality. It is not unusual at the pre-adolescent and adolescent stage for young people to develop "crushes" on members of the same sex, either adults or members of a peer group. Such "crushes" are normal and are usually resolved when the heterosexual stimulation overcomes the interest in this homosexual type of love relationship. The remnants of homosexuality are apparent in everyday behavior, and can be seen in adulthood, when strong friendships exist between two members of the same sex, for instance in membership in fraternal organizations, and even in such activities as an "evening spent with the boys," or a "card game with the girls." These are, however, natural minor counterparts of normal heterosexual behavior.

Homosexuality is difficult to diagnose in childhood, particularly in girls, because masculinity in girls is not as obvious as femininity in boys. Feminine behavior in boys, particularly on the elementary-school level, can take the form of a desire to dress up in female attire, put on lipstick, prefer a feminine role in a school play, or use perfume. They may even openly express their desire to be girls, and in such cases there is often a confusion in the use of pronouns. A boy who has strong conflicts in identification may refer to another boy as "she" without ever being aware of this confusion. Name-calling is quite prevalent among children, and those who are called "sissy" are frequently the physically undersized or the extremely passive ones who can be easily threatened by other children. Children who are called either "sissy," or in the case of girls, "tomboy," are not necessarily homosexual, but the possibility exists that they are deviates from their particular group at this particular time.

Boys are called "sissy" for several reasons: because they can't maintain their integrity by fighting; because they are interested in so-called "feminine" things, such as the arts; or because, in general, they assume a passive role. The "sissy" is abused because he cannot or will not engage in the acceptable activities of his peer group. Frequently, the "sissy" is the overly sensitive, highly intelligent child who is a deviate from his group only in the sense that he is a superior member of that group. The word "sissy" cannot be taken too seriously, unless a child gives many overt evidences of feminine behavior, or gives indications of some additional maladjustments. It is interesting to note that the boy who is called a "sissy" may suffer because of the derogatory implication, while a girl who is called a "tomboy" may, in our culture, enjoy the distinction of participating in boys' games, being accepted by boys, and being envied by girls for these special privileges.

In adolescence, the problem and conflict centering about peer acceptance, heterosexual activities, and identification, becomes greatly intensified. This is the period when homosexual adolescents begin to recognize themselves as deviates, and they look for others who are just like them. Adolescent homosexuals frequently leave home because they are unable to face the lack of parental understanding. They feel abused and mistreated, and in their search for security they look for a more benign environment away from home.

Most male homosexuals are overtly different and comparatively free in the expression of their needs. Many of them have adopted feminine traits which clearly mark them as deviate. The homosexual girl, however, has to be overtly deviate in dress and appearance before she is recognized. Unless she dresses in male clothing, cuts her hair in a mannish cut, refuses to wear make-up, and in other ways flagrantly imitates male behavior, she does not stand out as different. Adolescent girls who do not overtly imitate male behavior, and accept the feminine role, but only in relation to other females, cannot be detected as potential homosexuals unless other indications of maladjustment are so apparent that these girls are referred for psychological testing. It would then become evident that homosexuality is an integral part of the clinical picture and might be one of the underlying causes of the maladjustment.

Homosexual adolescents do not assume their deviant roles with comfortable ease. They recognize their differences, are aware that they are outcasts, and suffer because of it. The world does not accept them and they cannot accept themselves. While a young child does not understand or recognize potential homosexuality, although there may be an awareness of "being different" at a rather early age, the realization of the extent of the deviation does not have real import until adolescent sexual maturity is attained. This realization can be a tremendous shock because the homosexual, regardless of any insights, has been conditioned from early childhood to expect his development to parallel that of everyone else. This period of tragic realization is a particularly difficult stage in the life of an individual, and the stigma of homosexuality is so great that the adolescent is often afraid even to ask for help. The following essay, written by a homosexual boy, age 15, with an IQ exceeding 140, tells in poignant terms the meaning that his homosexuality has for him.

"The backgrounds of individuals affected by homosexuality are as varied as the individuals. On this topic, I would like to discuss my own background. From infancy on, I received too much love from my mother and nothing from my father. This was definitely not normal. Until the age of seven, I slept in the same room as my parents. Toilet training was given as discipline. I'm sure that self-regulation theories never even occurred to my parents. I was never given any freedom. My mother picked my friends and if she had her way she would be around to supervise my sexual activities. Luckily, she wasn't. She would have been shocked. I had excellent tutors in the really important matters like sex and bed manners, fencing, and whatever behavior goes into being a cultured gentleman on the continent. At eight and a half or nine, I slept with a fellow for the first time. When I was fifteen I first tried to sleep with a woman. It wasn't until her that I decided that this kind of love-making is plain cold sex. The fellow I'm going with now brought me to the conclusion that at least four hours of love play is necessary. I read that somewhere in *Love without Fear*. One of the most important factors that goes into the making of a gay kid is the love of finesse. Bed manners are not merely animal sex. Sex must come last. In enjoyment, it is the idea of love that matters."

It is apparent from this boy's writing that he is an extremely intelligent individual who has tried to find an explanation for his own deviation. He had read psychological books and had tried to gain insight into his behavior. In other words, he recognized that he needed help, but he always failed to find it. He continues to write as follows:

"I am part of the homosexual group, a group which is made to feel outcast in a so-called progressive society. The homosexual is referred to as 'gay' from the French *gaie*, even though they are perhaps the most miserable bunch of people in the world. Outwardly and to all appearances they are a happy, frivolous lot. They come from richest and poorest homes. Sex knows no differences and no class distinctions.

"They have one thing in common; their parents just don't understand it. They come from homes in which they are taught practically from infancy that gay people are horrible, or from homes in which sex is completely ignored. They come from every walk of life, and those who come from small towns are always heading to big cities where they hope to find friends and be more readily accepted. When they are not accepted by society, some manage to accept their fate, while others attempt to turn straight and in the process crack up. Some indulge in 'front' marriages (the lucky ones who are bisexual), but this doesn't make good adjustment. Some commit suicide and some identify with an organization such as the International Congress for Sexuality in order to attempt to change their fate.

"The lot of the gay kid is not a happy one. Most gay kids start surprisingly early in life. Some kids I've met claim to have been in bed with older men as early as the age of five. Unluckily, it seems that desire does not diminish with potency. Men over fifty and even over eighty and ninety still frequent the bars that are used by homosexuals, and it is due to these characters that homosexual prostitution is rampant.

"In homosexuality, religious and racial barriers do not exist. Members of both white and Negro circles are accepted by each other, and religion among 'gay kids' is what it should be among all people, a highly personal matter.

"The homosexual group is such an outcast group that it has developed a special esoteric language. An entire dictionary could be composed of the language used by homosexuals. The following gives merely a briefing on elemental language.

"An overtly feminine gay boy is called a 'queen' or a "swish,' while the one who appears masculine is called a 'butch queen,' differentiated from the one who actually assumes a man's role in the relationship who is called a 'butch.' A gay girl is called a 'dike' or 'dyke' from the story of the little Dutch boy who plugged up the hole in the wall with his finger. A masculine dike is a 'bull dagger' or 'bull diker,' while a feminine one is merely a 'fem dike.' 'Browning' is anal intercourse, and '69' is mutual fellatio. The performance of the equivalent of fellatio anally is called 'rimming.' To 'camp' is to swish in the hopes of 'making' someone, while to 'cruise' is considered to be 'on the make.' A 'tearoom' is a men's room used for 'cruising.'"

This boy evidently had a real awareness of his conflict at a very early age. His school record indicated that he showed symptoms of maladjustment in the classroom, even while there seemed to be no overt manifestation of feminine behavior. He was small for his age, undernourished and sickly, and had a record of many absences which later developed into truancy. His record states that he came from a home in which the mother assumed the masculine role, working and supporting the family, while the father, who was in ailing health, remained at home to keep house. He had an intense distrust of adults and his teachers felt he was always suspicious of their motives. As he matured into adolescence, he looked to the school for help by asking rather pointed questions regarding psychological deviation in the sexual areas. His search for help from the school was unsuccessful and he became a chronic truant. It is, of course, questionable as to what kind of help would have really been of much assistance to a boy like this. Even psychological therapy and psychoanalysis have been able to do little more than assist homosexuals to accept their homosexuality, and to keep them from getting into conflict with the law.

SUMMARY

Sex deviations are part of the broader problem of maladjustments. They may appear in all diagnostic categories: psychosis, neurosis, or simple behavior problems. Certain types of sex deviations are apparent in overt behavior and are expressed in the classroom in the form of obscenities, excessive sex play, masturbation and, occasionally, sex-role confusion. The teacher should regard this type of symptomatology not as bad conduct which is flagrantly disrespectful, but, rather, as guide-posts to detecting and understanding the nature of disturbed behavior.

Chapter VII

The Psychopathic Personality

An exact definition has yet to be given of the meaning of the diagnostic label *psychopath*. In clinical terminology it is not synonymous with either psychosis, neurosis, or simple maladjustment, but seems rather to be a specific syndrome of maladjustive behavior which does not fall into any other category. It is a pattern of behavior resulting from a specific etiology and is one of the most difficult forms of disturbance to detect without psychological investigation. The psychopath is an individual who, in simplified terms, has no "conscience." Psychopaths have a common developmental history which indicates that, in the first two years of life, they have been deprived of a mother and of any consistent affection by a mother substitute. These children never function well in affectional relationships, and never having experienced love, are not really aware of its existence.

Psychopaths are concerned with self-love and in meeting their own needs regardless of how this affects others. They are interested in self-gratification and adopt any means, right or wrong, to gain their ends. Intellectually they know the difference between moral and immoral acts, but emotionally they are incapable of responding to the rightness or wrongness of an act, never investing their behavior with any emotional content. When they commit acts which they know are wrong intellectually, they experience no emotional pressure, anxiety, or feelings of guilt. These are the children who may steal, lie, or cheat without feeling that it is wrong to do so. When they are punished, they show no real sorrow, chagrin, or unhappiness, and when it suits their purposes, they engage in the same previously punished, antisocial behavior all over again. They do not learn from experience, and are interested only in the pursuit of their own goals. These are the children who can be dangerous to the community, because they have no guilt or remorse. Many psychopathic children are extremely charming, bright, and delightful, but they cannot make good relationships with people except on a very superficial level. They never have close friends and do not relate to the adults in the environment. They maneuver people and situations to suit their own needs and demand attention which they usually receive because of their great superficial charm. Psychopaths can "turn the charm on or off" at will, however, and even when an adult feels that a good relationship has been established, time will show that none exists.

The psychopath can abuse, at any moment, the very person from whom he has derived the greatest benefits. He is completely feelingless except in relation to his own desires, being amoral rather than immoral, and asocial rather than antisocial. The world exists only for him, and he has no concern about the welfare of others. Unless he engages in a really destructive act, there may be no awareness by others of the severity of his personality deviation. The psychopath is really dangerous in that he can engage in criminal acts, sexual delinquencies, drug addiction, or in any other form of unacceptable activity which interests him without any recognition of right or wrong.

Lois E.: Female, Age 12, IQ 92

At birth, Lois was put in an institution because her mother was a prostitute. The mother returned when Lois was two and provided a home for her, but she continued to engage in prostitution. Lois was subsequently placed in several foster homes, until the age of eight, when she returned to live with her mother. During her stay in foster homes, Lois was never able to get along. She was a constant truant from school, and ran away from every foster home several times. She had friends, but liked to engage in isolated activities, reading, going alone to the movies, etc. She was eventually brought to a psychiatric hospital for constant truanting from school, for running away from home, and for suspicion of stealing.

The psychological tests revealed an inability to identify with people and a lack of emotional attachments. She had a vivid phantasy life where she had ideas of being happy, popular and loved. Her judgments were exceedingly poor in that she was interested only in pursuing her own goals without giving any regard to the needs of other people. She gave no indication of anxiety in situations where realistic anxiety should have been evidenced. The diagnosis read, "character disorder with psychopathic trends." It was predicted that this girl would develop into a full-blown psychopath.

Andrew F.: Male, Age 15, IQ 89

Andrew was a foundling who was placed, when only a few hours old, at a church door. Because he was very ill immediately after birth (it appeared most likely that he was premature at birth), Andrew was placed in an institutional hospital setting. There he remained for the first nine months of his life. At nine months, he was placed in a foster home, but a severe pneumonia returned him to the hospital for another month. When Andrew was ready for release from the hospital, the foster home he had been in was not available, and Andrew was returned to the foundling institution. He remained there until the age of sixteen months when he was placed again. After three months of being in the new foster home, the foster parent died and Andrew was again returned to the institution. This time he remained there until he was two years of age. Again he was placed in a home where he remained until he was five. At that time, Andrew's behavior became a source of difficulty at home. On one occasion, he locked a younger foster sister in the bathroom. At another time, he pushed a neighbor's child down a flight of stairs. He had frequent temper tantrums at home and in nursery school. When Andrew tried to set fire to the mattress, his foster mother reluctantly gave him up. Then began a series of placements for Andrew, none of which proved successful. In ten years, Andrew was tried in thirteen different homes. He failed in each of them. His aggressive behavior became more overt as he grew older. He consistently stole money, truanted from school, and ran away, presumably to get to Hollywood. Occasionally he set fires. At the age of fifteen, he was sent for psychiatric observation when he caused several thousand dollars worth of damage in his attempt to burn down his school.

Psychiatric evaluation revealed an inability to identify with any meaningful person in the environment. He had no concept of himself or of his role in society. Because there had been no stable relationship in his early years, he had not been capable of identifying with an adult figure. Thus, Andrew could not see himself in an adult role. Authority had no meaning to him, his disregard of it being represented by his asocial behavior. Andrew was remarkably free from anxiety, indicating that his own behavior was viewed by him as acceptable. Andrew was incapable, therefore, of understanding the concepts of right and wrong, not because he did not want to, but because his past history was such that he could no longer develop the concepts in more than a superficial manner.

SUMMARY

The psychopathic personality is defined as a clinical entity, unrelated to any other form of disturbance. The term *psychopathic* refers in lay terms to any individual who is asocial, shiftless, irresponsible, and undisciplined. In psychological terminology, *psychopath* refers to those individuals who, when on good behavior, are attractive, ingratiating, highly entertaining, and charming, but who are incapable, however, of investing a relationship with adequate emotionality. When pursuing their own goals, they can become vicious, offensive, and criminal. Their own needs are of paramount importance and they are bent on self-gratification without any feelings of guilt, anxiety, sorrow, or emotional pain. They are completely self-centered and have no regard for the environment. They do not care to change their behavior, being perfectly content with what they are. Even when they seem to make the effort to reform, the promise is forgotten before a few minutes are past. They are controlled by, "I want, I must have," and they behave accordingly. Typical of psychopathic behavior is an incident reported in a newspaper about a man who, charged with passing a bad check, appeared before the judge and promised to "go straight." He then promptly paid his fine with a worthless check.

Chapter VIII

The Teacher and the Disturbed Child*

Education is an essential and vital element in the life and growth of every child. In our society, nothing is more important to a child than to be able to get along, somehow, in a classroom situation. Unless he is given the help necessary to enable him to function in school, everything else that is done for him is just not enough. If he is to live with any degree of adequacy, a child must learn to get along in a classroom.

Education today stresses child growth, emotionally, socially, and academically. In these terms, education cannot be construed merely as teaching children how to read, write, and do arithmetic. There has been a gradual change in primary emphasis from academic subjects to the child himself, his experiences, and his needs. Subject matter and skills, of course, must be taught, but in relation to and as natural outcomes of children's experiences and their changing needs.

The disturbed child comes to school with many needs and very few good experiences. Whether he is placed in a regular class, an adjustment class, or a special class for disturbed children, he reacts to the school situation with hostility, suspicion, reluctance, and frustration.

---

*The material in this chapter is based in part upon the following articles written by the authors: "A Method of Establishing Rapport with the Disturbed Child," *Understanding the Child*, Vol. XXI, No. 1 (January, 1952); "The Dynamics of Need-Acceptance Relationships for the Emotionally Disturbed Child in the Classroom," *The Nervous Child*, Vol. 10, No. 3-4 (1954); and "Remedial Reading for the Disturbed Child," *Clearing House*, Vol. 30, No. 3 (November, 1955).

School is a problem for this child and this child is a problem for the school. If he has been in school previously, his cumulative record is a semantic nightmare of unflattering adjectives, such as "insolent," "incorrigible," "unmanageable," "indifferent," "antisocial," "lazy," and "shy." However, he has been labeled, and whatever the implications of his behavior, one thing is clearly evident; he is an unhappy child. He is driven by undesirable impulses which he either expresses directly, endangering the environment, or represses, causing injury to himself. Both of these means leave his needs unsatisfied, increase his emotional tensions, and serve only to help perpetuate his faulty functioning.

It is no small task for the teacher to keep this child. There are certain common practices and procedures, however, which can aid the teacher in classroom situations regardless of whether the teacher is concerned with one disturbed child among a group of thirty or with a class of disturbed children in a treatment center.

THE TEACHER AND NEED-ACCEPTANCE THERAPY

A basic precept for the establishment of a good working teacher-pupil relationship is the theory of acceptance. A child has to learn to accept the teacher and the school situation. The teacher, in turn, must accept the child along with the manifestations of his difficulties. This acceptance begins the moment the child enters the classroom. The initial contact with the child lays the foundation for all future relations, and may make the difference between a teaching failure and a teaching success.

The first few days are days of orientation during which the teacher notes and tries to understand the child's behavior. This is the time, also, when the child tests the limits of his acceptability and the limits of the teacher's patience.

School cannot be "crammed" down the child's throat. The active relationships between the pupil and the teacher and among the pupil and his peers are more important at this time than the acquisition of the academic tools of learning. A teacher cannot aim for academic remediation until there has been an increase in social adaptability and a willingness to submit to assistance. The first rung on the ladder of academic learning is climbed when the child accepts the teacher and the teacher accepts the child.

Every school has the responsibility for providing the practical means to encourage this acceptance. Formal restrictions can be relaxed to alleviate some of the anxiety the child associates with school. The non-competitive, friendly atmosphere of a good living place which permits individuality and self-expression provides a therapeutic school situation.

The teacher in this setting can provide realistic educational goals for those who are deficient or blocked. Special teaching methods geared to the individual must be constantly re-evaluated to clarify individual differences and to maintain the balance between environmental needs and developmental changes.

Every classroom, however, is concerned not only with the individual, but of necessity with the group as well. When working with a group of disturbed children, or with a disturbed child in a group of normal children, the teacher must provide the child with adequate working experiences throughout the day.

The atmosphere in the classroom should be permissive and the program elastic enough to ensure that each child is reached on his own level of development. The classroom should present a picture of diverse activities in which the disturbed child can work on his own project, academic or nonacademic, secure in the knowledge that what he is doing is looked upon with approval and is of value to himself and to the group. The function of the teacher is to provide experiences which the child can meet with growing confidence and success.

In such a classroom one child may be drawing, another doing woodwork, and a third typing, while the rest of the class may be engaged in a group activity. There may even be a child who is apparently unoccupied. This child may be adjusting to the classroom situation and to the teacher. The "doing nothingness" state of his growth may be just a phase of development, and being part of this group without destroying it, may well be the learning achievement for this pupil. The "doing nothingness" may represent intensive work on the part of the teacher, who has guided him to the point where he is willing to be in the room without being unruly and destructive. No matter what developmental stage has been reached with each child in that room, the teacher has worked with that child and has accepted him as an individual.

When working with the emotionally disturbed child, the teacher acts as the person who provides a benign therapeutic environment which will permit the child to express his emotions, whatever they may be, without censure; to control these emotions realistically within the framework of what is considered socially acceptable; and to provide him with opportunities for possible insight into his own behavior.

The setting of this educative stage is a slow and difficult process. The child evaluates and re-evaluates the teacher, who is constantly providing him with opportunities to express himself with work which is well within his narrow limitations. The child begins to realize that the teacher is able to create for him a salutary environment in which he may begin to function adequately, but despite this realization, he may still be hostile and unaccepting of the authoritarian role of the teacher. The relationship which the teacher is constantly trying to build and which the child seems to want to dissolve is almost a tangible one. When the child feels secure enough with this relationship so that he stops testing it, real adjustment begins.

The teacher's role, therefore, is a difficult one. The role of teacher-academician concerned with skills and discipline has given way to a new concept of teaching concerned with education of the emotions. In order to accomplish this goal, the teacher has to accept the behavior of the child from his first moment in class, no matter how unacceptable that behavior may be. The disturbed child who is aggressive is permitted to express his aggression without harming himself or others, while the withdrawn child is not pressured into socializing, but is treated with intelligent neglect. Every child is made to feel that the teacher accepts him as an individual and that his behavior will be met with understanding. Because this is such an unusual role for a teacher to assume, the disturbed child meets the teacher with great suspicion and hostility. He will attempt at every opportunity to test the limits of the teacher's patience. The teacher, while trying to break down the child's concept of authority as a threatening force, maintains a constant emotional climate of returning good for evil. Little by little, the child begins to realize that perhaps nothing he can do will break the relationship, while at the same time he becomes aware that his behavior is considered socially unacceptable. The teacher makes it quite clear that no matter what the child does, he is accepted and liked as an individual.

The following description of Alex, and the way the teacher reacted to Alex's behavior, is an example of how one disturbed child began to improve:

Alex, age eleven, was an extremely aggressive child who engaged in violent temper tantrums whenever he could not dominate the situation. When he walked into the classroom for the first time, he was sullen and obstreperous and seemed aware of the fact that he was considered unacceptable. He felt himself to be different from other people. He was "killed with love" by all the staff who had contact with him in school. The affection was not insincere however, for Alex, like most children, was quick to sense an unreal situation, particularly so when he was the focus of the unreality. Approbation could not be given to his cruel acts, but he was praised lavishly and made to feel essential and secure in the classroom at every small opportunity.

The turning point in Alex's behavior was reached after he had indulged in a particularly stormy temper tantrum and had flung jars of paints over the room. He was not punished, however, but merely asked to mop the floor and repair the damage. His final challenge had not succeeded in making the teacher reprimand him. He was faced, for the first time in his school history, perhaps, with a situation he could not continue to handle in an aggressive fashion, for it no longer gained him prestige to be the class bully. As Alex felt that he was always accepted by the teacher, and as in acceptance lay security, he could no longer endanger that security by acting in a hostile manner. In addition, the teacher, by providing him with an atmosphere of warmth and understanding, let him know that the same feeling was expected from him in return. Alex could not tolerate the guilt feelings within him each time he felt the teacher had been the target of his aggression. To alleviate his guilt, he felt the need to conform. In conformity lay acceptance. This was met with praise and approval, and because it netted him greater emotional satisfaction than had his former aggression, his outward manifestations of maladjustment began to decrease.

Alex began to struggle with a first-year reader, do arithmetic, and work diligently at copying spelling words from the blackboard. He asked for academic work. For the first time in his school career he was a conformist.

His bullying practices were diverted into constructive activities, and he even began to help others apply themselves to academic endeavors.

The growth in Alex's maturity was not smooth and steady. There were temporary setbacks and uncontrollable sieges of temper while learning how to control tempestuous emotions. One factor, however, remained constant—he was always certain that the teacher accepted him as an individual, even though there was disapproval of his behavior at any given time. His behavior may have been frowned upon, but never Alex himself. These were two separate entities. In essence, that is the philosophy which makes this practice of acceptance a workable one. The story of Alex can be repeated many times over with many different children, each one responding in his own way to the teacher, and each one adjusting to the school situation with a degree of social success never heretofore enjoyed by him in the classroom.

During the process of emotional adjustment, the child may manipulate the teacher into certain roles, depending upon his needs at the moment. The teacher may assume the role of the idealized parent figure, petting and cuddling the child upon demand. It is hardly unusual for a disturbed nine- or ten-year-old child to crawl onto the teacher's lap and demand warm physical comfort. The child is thus ascribing to the teacher a role which he phantasies, and which allows him to satisfy his own infantile needs. If this is the part the child wants the teacher to assume, the teacher must be ready to meet him on this level at this particular time. William, for example, was a nine-year-old boy who was placed in a special class for disturbed children because of excessive truancy in the regular grades. This boy was extremely quiet when he first came into class. He would not participate in the activities of the group. He looked for direction in everything he did, seeking constant approval and reassurance. He would not try new materials until he spent time observing others using them. Even activities which were familiar to him appeared to be threatening. He could not color a picture, for instance, without asking what colors to use and checking and rechecking to make certain the color was correct. When coloring a bird, for instance, he asked, "What color should it be? Is yellow a good color?" When he was told that yellow was fine, he continued with, "Is yellow a good color? Are you sure birds are yellow? Do you like yellow?" These questions went on endlessly, until the activity was completed, at which time he asked, ad infinitum, "Did I do good? Do you like it, teacher? Is yellow good? Do you think it's good?"

This boy, of course, was suffering from a deep sense of personal inadequacy. His lack of self-esteem stemmed from emotional deprivation in his early years. He was certain no one loved him, not even his mother. He was convinced, moreover, that no one could like him, because he considered himself as unlikable, unworthy of love and affection. And yet he sought this love in every relationship he made. Unfortunately, even as he sought love he also repelled others from liking him. His constant nagging questions were a source of irritation to others; children as well as most adults in his home environment rebuffed him. And so the love he sought by this demanding behavior was refused him because of the very offensive quality of the behavior itself.

William constantly haunted the teacher with his endless questions of reassurance. As many times as the questions were asked, however, they were given an answer. Time after time the teacher reassured him of his own skill in doing an activity. Gradually, William began to believe in himself, and gradually his questions began to decrease in intensity and quality. With this decrease, however, William's behavior began to change subtly. As his relationship with his teacher became more and more supportive to him, he became more and more overtly affectionate. One day he held her hand. Another day, he put an arm around her waist. A third day he even kissed her. And then, quite without warning, as the teacher was sitting at the desk working with him individually on an arithmetic problem, he slid onto her lap. The teacher accepted this without comment, and went on explaining the lesson. The rest of the lesson continued in this way. This behavior began to occur more frequently as time went on. Upon occasion, William called her "mama" without seeming to know he had done so.

The teacher was always ready to accept William's need for this kind

Rue:

Thanks —

12/2/63

Alice Wheeler
Bee Sarte — Montevlado — Ul...

of mothering. Sometimes just by her accepting attitudes William knew he was liked. Upon occasion, however, the teacher would verbalize her affection for him. The following conversation reflects her acceptance of William's emotional needs and his growing insight into his own behavior:

TEACHER: I had a little boy once just about your size. He used to sit on my lap, too.
WILLIAM: Was his name William?
TEACHER: No, it wasn't.
WILLIAM: Did you like him?
TEACHER: Yes—and I like you.
WILLIAM: Did you hold him on your lap?
TEACHER: Yes, like I'm holding you.
WILLIAM: Do you like me?
TEACHER: Yes, I love you.
WILLIAM: I love you, too.
TEACHER: You like to pretend you're my baby.
WILLIAM: Yes. (Cuddling closer.)
TEACHER: You would like to be a little baby.
WILLIAM: Yes.
TEACHER: I love you when you're a little baby. Everybody likes to be a baby sometimes, but it's more fun being grown up. Babies can't be monitors and give out paper, but big boys can. Would you like to? (*William quickly jumped out of her lap, went to the paper closet, and began distributing paper.*)

It is evident from this conversation that the teacher understood and accepted the role that William imposed on her. Even while she played this role, she was guiding him into more mature patterns. The process, of course, was a slow one, but William did gain insights into his own emotional needs. As the term went on the frequency with which he exhibited this infantile behavior diminished.

At another time, perhaps, the teacher acts as a buffer and protects the child from his inadequacies, even to the point of assuming blame for a given situation. The child may accuse the teacher of being the cause of his failure in an activity. A child who in frustration tears a page out of a reader may turn upon the teacher, accusing the teacher of his failure. When the teacher seemingly agrees with the child, recognizes his feelings and reflects them back to him, the tension is relieved. In this way, if the teacher assumes the guilt and accepts the blame for the failure, the child is relieved of the responsibility for his own inadequacies and is ready to try again. The teacher may at this time also stress the universality of the feeling expressed by the child, giving the child the understanding that he is not alone either in the emotion experienced or in the situation which gave rise to the difficulty. This kind of discussion with a child frequently involves other children in the group with the result that this child is provided with greater security because he recognizes that he is not isolated.

When Helen, for example, a compulsive, anxious girl of eleven, burst into uncontrollable crying because she was unable to do a division example, the teacher apologized for the situation by saying, "Oh, I made a mistake. I picked an example from the wrong book. It's all my fault. I must be stupid today. Give me the paper, I'll put an example on it from the right book."

Helen stopped her crying immediately and said, "You're not stupid, teacher." The teacher replied, "Oh yes, everybody is stupid sometime."

Charlie, who was sitting on the other side of the room apparently oblivious to the situation, suddenly called out, "That's right. Me too. Once I came to school with two different shoes on. That was stupid."

And Jose chimed in at this point, saying, "Me, I'm a lot stupid—I get on the wrong bus going home and I go somewhere else instead and I get home late and my mother she calls me stupid."

As these confessions were elicited, Helen's smile became more pronounced and she busily resettled herself with different examples. Her anxiety was dissipated by this exchange of feelings and she was able to continue.

Upon other occasions, a child may manipulate the teacher into the role of a peer. At these times, he expects the teacher to respond to him as a child might. The teacher then operates at the child's emotional and perceptual level. The teacher may indulge in colloquial speech patterns, meeting the child with his own language and responding and participating with enthusiasm in the child's activities.

In a recreation period, for instance, the teacher might run races with the children, play jacks, shoot marbles, wheel the doll carriage, or in other ways participate actively in the children's play. In speaking on the child's own level, the teacher may respond to the child's, "Hey, teach!" with, "Hey, kid!" This kind of repartee frequently alleviates stress situations in a classroom. The following situation is an example of how a teacher can redirect hostility and establish the tenor of the class so that children can function with emotional comfort:

Richard's paper was accidentally knocked off his desk by Lillian. Richard exploded with, "You bitch, pick that up."
Lillian answered, "You bitch, I will not."
Richard repeated, "You bitch, you betta."
The teacher said, "Bitch, bitch. Stop bitching. I'll pick it up." Whereupon the teacher picked up the paper and the children proceeded with their work.

The teacher's acceptance of the word without moralizing and her own use of the word acted as a calming influence on the children in that emphasizing the word "bitch" in an ordinary casual way de-emphasized the emotional implications.

This same procedure applied with caution is frequently effective in handling situations in which children use obscene language. The teacher's acceptance and use of an obscenity takes the shock effect away from the word so that it loses its aggressive connotations and its value as an attention-getting mechanism.

Frequently, the teacher can become a subservient figure who can be bullied and made to serve the ego needs of the child. In assuming this role, the teacher helps the aggressive child become less anxious, guiding his aggression, thereby preventing this aggression from falling upon other children. When it seems necessary, therefore, to acquiesce to a child's unreasonable aggressive demands, the teacher must be willing to do so. In most cases, when this child, little by little, becomes aware that his demands are being met, he also becomes more willing to relinquish them, and begins to function with less hostility and unreasonableness.

Not only does the teacher sometimes have to assume a subservient role, but conversely, she may also, at other times, become the hero figure, the great defender who protects the child from all evil. Some children find it too difficult to participate in group activities because of their own inadequacies or because of a reality situation which is overpowering. Such a child looks to the teacher for protection and for assistance in establishing his own status in the group. The teacher may then become the omnipotent force who, all powerful, makes a pleasant classroom world for the child.

The teacher has a relationship differing in quality and intensity with each child, and each child accepts the teacher in any role which the moment demands either with him or with another child. Children see no incongruity in the fact that the teacher can be so many things to so many children. Within each of these roles, however, the teacher maintains an identity related to the classroom structure; the role momentarily assumed is superimposed upon everyday classroom routine. The reality situation is actually never lost and the child recognizes this fact even while he may overtly deny it.

For many children it is a unique experience to find that they are able to manage their emotions with the help of a teacher who not only understands their needs, but who is responsive to them in an active, supportive manner. No progress, of course, is without setbacks. There are times when the teacher cannot clearly determine the role the child wishes her to play. If the assumed role is not the one the child intended, the teacher must discard it. In such cases, the child does not respond to the role, resists it, denies it, or perhaps is merely amused by it. He may remark, "You're silly," "Come off it," "I don't want to be a baby," "Let me alone," or "Cut it out, teach." It is reassuring to know that roles incorrectly assumed or wrong interpretations are in no way damaging to the child. The child exercises his prerogative to reject them, and the teacher must try again. Teaching for emotional adjustment continues until the child is able to function as an individual, with less and less recourse to the contrived experiences which the teacher has provided. The teacher then finds that the child becomes able to conform to group restrictions and authority regulations, and that gradually he can develop an inner self-discipline.

The following study of Jose, age ten, demonstrates most clearly how need-acceptance therapy can contribute to emotional adjustment. The case is presented in the teacher's own words in order to demonstrate not only the reactions of the teacher to the child, but also the reactions of the child to a specific situation, and the various roles the teacher felt she had to play in response to Jose's needs.

"Jose D. is a ten-year-old, white Puerto Rican boy who was admitted to the hospital * in October of 1953 because of frequent uncontrollable temper outbursts in which it was feared he might kill his mother. He was hyperactive and believed that his physical strength was superhuman. Prior to his admission, he had almost been killed in his attempt to control and stop traffic. He felt that he was stronger than the force of automobiles. He was disoriented and unaware of the fact that he was in a hospital.

"Jose had never attended school in Puerto Rico because of his severe emotional problems and his inability to conform. He could not read or write Spanish and he had no knowledge of English. He did not understand the simplest communication put to him.

"When Jose first came to this school he was completely unapproachable and bizarre. He made grimaces at me, made obscene gestures, laughed and talked to himself, threw furniture and paints, and in general was one of the most aggressive children ever to come into the ward. He refused any sort of contact with me, even throwing away the candy I offered him. He kept running out of the room into the gymnasium, pushing other children from the swings so that he himself could swing and try to fly. The only word he spoke was 'Superman.'

"His behavior continued to be erratic and bizarre until I approached him through the medium of art. I asked him to draw, but he refused. I myself then began to draw. I started a picture of Superman. A wide grin spread over his face and with a sign of approval he began to draw a red devil. We spent the day exchanging our pictures. For the next few days, our relationship consisted of drawing and showing each other what we had drawn. Jose painted and drew almost compulsively. He was very artistic and his paintings were most original and showed unusual merit. It was his first painting experience anywhere and Jose was delighted with it. He painted for days at a time, receiving constant approval, even though his themes were bizarre and macabre.

---

* The hospital referred to is a psychiatric hospital. The school which Jose attended while a patient at the hospital is situated within the hospital itself.

Surfeited - surfeit - N - excess - excess in eating or drinking -
- v - to supply with anything to excess or satiate — to indulge to excess in anything

"As he realized that I accepted his phantasy, he began to relate to me and to the children, and gradually he accepted the school situation. His phantasy life was his only interest. Using this interest, we began a phantasy booklet devoted to the topic, 'Things That Fly.' In this way, Jose began to learn how to read. He was very proud of his reader and showed it to all visitors. He began to extend his interests from Superman to more realistic flying things, and so we read and discussed the airplane, birds, etc. Jose was getting ready to relinquish his obsession and to experiment with the more realistic world.

"During this period, I read to Jose at every opportunity. He stopped his constant painting and climbed onto my lap to listen to stories. He was now able to differentiate between his phantasy and reality. He began to read and to express an interest in academic work.

"Jose has now made a remarkable academic, social, and emotional adjustment. He is reading a first-grade book. He speaks English fluently. He no longer runs into the gymnasium, and prefers to spend his time either reading or playing a quiet game with the children. His paintings are less bizarre.

"Jose's improvement was so dramatic that the doctors felt he should continue attending this school as long as possible. Special provision was made whereby Jose's stay at the hospital could continue indefinitely, and he could continue to make progress."

It is clear from the teacher's account of Jose's behavior that she was able to work with Jose only on the basis of accepting his behavior for what it was. She did not try to change him initially, but rather accepted him on the level, bizarre as it was, on which he was functioning. It is also clear that most of the time was spent playing the role of a peer, entering his phantasy life much as another child might, and responding to him in a childlike manner. It was only when Jose was surfeited with this relationship and with his own phantasy that he was able to relinquish both the relationship and the phantasy for more mature patterns of functioning.

As demonstrated by the illustrative material, need-acceptance therapy in the classroom is teacher recognition of the propelling dynamic forces of child behavior, and the acceptance of that behavior on all levels whether expressed in destructive, negative, hostile, and aggressive terms, or in withdrawn, isolated, and passive behavior. In response to the child's behavior, the teacher assumes the various role characteristics that are imposed as they arise from the child's emotional needs. The teacher, thereby, affords each child a need-acceptance relationship which is not analytical although it can be reflective and may be interpretive. It exists simply to permit the child to work through his tensions, phantasies, regressions, and hostilities with the teacher in the classroom, thus helping the child to greater emotional maturity.

Need-acceptance in the classroom is teacher acceptance of the principle that the learning process involves not only the acquisition of academic skills, but also the acquisition of social values. Self-respect on the part of the pupil for his own individual worth, recognition of the worth of others, and respect for the rights of others are important aspects of this learning. In this educative process, academic achievement becomes a secondary goal. The primary goal of the teacher is to help the child gain a personal evaluation of himself and to attain an emotional adjustment.

Who Should Teach the Disturbed Child?

The teacher of the disturbed child should be a strange, hybrid creature who is emotionally mature, well grounded in education and psychology, talented in the arts, has a wide range of interests, and with all these attributes is aware of personal limitations. Teachers who are most successful with disturbed children are genuine human beings who have insights into their own needs and have the capacity to become an integral part of a treatment team.

It is not feasible, of course, to make a list of all the possible insights and understandings which a teacher of emotionally disturbed children should possess. However, the following outline represents an effort to clarify certain very basic understandings which a successful teacher must accept. It suggests, in relation both to others and to oneself, a frame of reference for developing the insights necessary for effective teaching with disturbed children.

The teacher must realize that:

1. *The disturbed child is not* unwilling *to conform; he is, essentially,* unable *to conform.*
2. *The disturbed child must be permitted to speak out in anger without being harshly censured. The teacher who reacts aggressively to aggressive behavior is satisfying her own needs, not the needs of the child. There is no contradiction here, however, in terms of ag-*

gressive responses, when a child manipulates the teacher into a role. At this time, the teacher is not personally experiencing emotion, merely assuming emotion for therapeutic reasons. When, however, the teacher actually becomes emotionally involved with a child, the teacher is meeting her own personal needs and is not concerned with those of the child.

3. The disturbed child has uneven patterns of development and the teacher must accept these patterns, teaching not by a required curriculum, but in terms of emotional needs.

4. The disturbed child is frequently impulsive, disorganized, aggressive, and negativistic. He must not be sacrificed to meet the teacher's need for order, conformity, and passivity.

5. The teacher's need is not necessarily the child's need. If fulfillment comes only from seeing academic learning take place, the teacher is not prepared to work therapeutically with the disturbed child. If superiority as a teacher means insisting upon the acquisition of academic knowledge and skills, no success with the disturbed child is possible.

6. The teacher's interest in a child must not be a morbid one, or one in which the teacher becomes too deeply involved emotionally. Therapy can take place only when the teacher is an impartial, sympathetic observer, not an emotionally involved participant.

7. The teacher must not use teaching the disturbed child as a means of resolving personal problems. However, with insight into personal problems the teacher can understand and evaluate them and thereby prevent them from interfering with the treatment and therapy of the child.

8. The impulsive behavior of the disturbed child must be channelized into spontaneous fun which offers this child more appropriate realistic experiences than unsuccessful attempts at formal academic achievement.

9. The teacher must recognize symptoms and be continually aware of subliminal communication as a tool for true understanding. The teacher must know that all communication does not have to be verbalized.

Chapter IX

Personality Projection Through Verbal Expression

PROJECTION TECHNIQUES

Clinical assessment of personality refers to an evaluation of a battery of tests administered by a trained psychologist. The psychologist gives a series of tests designed to explore the significant emotional and mental characteristics of an individual. The psychologist is interested in determining the level of intellectual functioning, potential capacity, basic conflicts, and manner in which these conflicts are resolved. The psychological battery usually includes tests of personality and intelligence, and very often also includes tests of interests, aptitude, and achievement. The psychologist takes all the information provided by the tests, and integrates and interprets them in order to obtain an evaluation of the way an individual is functioning. The purpose of this evaluation is to obtain the basic patterns an individual uses to adjust to the testing situations, and, in interpreting these patterns, predict future behavior and the degree of ultimate adjustment.

In personality evaluation, it is important to know the level of intelligence at which the individual is actually functioning. In assessing intelligence in children, the two tests most frequently used are the Revised Edition of the Stanford-Binet, Forms L and M;[1] and the Wechsler

---

[1] L. Terman and M. Merrill, *Measuring Intelligence, a Guide to the Administration of the New Revised Stanford-Binet Tests of Intelligence* (New York: Houghton Mifflin, 1937).

Intelligence Scale for Children.[2] These tests are primarily effective for school-age children from five through adolescence. For very young children, scales of maturational development, such as compiled by Gesell,[3] are most frequently used as measures of intelligence.

The assessment of personality is a much more difficult task than the measurement of intelligence. In this area, several determinations must be made. Is the individual who takes the test reacting normally to his environment so that he may be considered fairly well adjusted? Is he functioning on a neurotic level and therefore must he be considered disturbed? Is he psychotic, and if so, what is the nature of his psychosis? Certainly, even within these three very broad categories, there are many possibilities of variation in the levels and types of functioning or malfunctioning.

In order to provide the psychologist with the necessary information for personality evaluation, certain clinical tools have been developed which are known as projective tests of personality.

The word *projection* still remains to be defined in a manner acceptable to all psychologists who are semantically concerned. There is, however, general acceptance of certain meanings inherent in the psychological context of the word. *Projection* was first used in a psychological sense by Freud, who referred to a defensive mechanism which permitted the individual to release or project upon the environment internal ideational and emotional processes.[4]

Frank was the first one to use the term *projective technique,* defining projective tests as those in which the individual projects ". . . patterns or configurations upon widely different materials and reveals in his life history the sequence of experiences that make these projections psychologically meaningful for his personality." [5]

In Warren's *Dictionary of Psychology,* projection is defined as ". . .

---

[2] D. Wechsler, *Wechsler Intelligence Scale for Children* (New York: Psychological Corporation, 1949).

[3] A. Gesell, *Studies in Child Development* (New York: Harper & Brothers, 1948).

[4] Sigmund Freud, *The Basic Writings of Sigmund Freud,* ed. A. A. Brill (New York: Random House, 1938), p. 857.

[5] L. K. Frank, "Projective Methods for the Study of Personality," *Journal of Psychology,* VIII (1939), 389–413.

the tendency to ascribe to the external world repressed mental processes which are not recognized as being of personal origin and as a result of which the content of these processes is experienced as an outer perception." Noyes, in essential agreement with this definition, states that in using the mechanism of projection, the individual casts out from his internal awareness his own unacceptable feelings, and places them upon other persons in the environment.[6] In doing so, the individual attempts to free himself from his own anxiety in dealing with these unacceptable feelings.

In evaluating the definitions of projection, Bell states that the elements common to the various definitions of projection are that ". . . the process of projection is unconscious, that it serves as a defense against unconscious impulses, feelings, ideas, and attitudes, and finally, that it reduces personal tension." [7] It would appear, then, that in personality projection the "subject manifests his personality . . . by 'thrusting it out' where it may be inspected. In the 'throwing' the personality is not grossly modified; it is only externalized in behavior that is typical of the individual." [8]

Although projective techniques are widely used by psychologists in private practice, in psychiatric clinics and hospitals, and in child guidance centers, the hypotheses underlying the interpretation of projective tests have not as yet been proved to everyone's satisfaction. For instance, some tests of personality evaluation, such as the Rorschach, have not been statistically validated. There has, however, been empirical validation of the test (research studies in the Rorschach technique far outnumber the studies devoted to any other projective test).

The Rorschach test is certainly one of the most widely used of all projective techniques. To administer, score, and interpret it properly requires years of intensive study, not only of the test itself, but of personality theory. The psychologist must be able, in the light of his findings on the Rorschach, to relate these conclusions to personality development and theory.

---

[6] A. P. Noyes, *Modern Clinical Psychiatry* (Philadelphia: W. B. Saunders Co., 1934).

[7] J. Bell, *Protective Techniques* (New York: Longmans, Green & Co., 1948), p. 2.

[8] *Ibid.*, p. 3.

The Rorschach test is named after Hermann Rorschach, a Swiss psychiatrist who endeavored to discover a practical method of differential diagnosis. His work, *Psychodiagnostik*,[9] published in 1921, consists of a series of ten ink blots and a discussion of how the test should be administered, scored, and interpreted. His work was so monumental and so brilliant in concept that, to a great extent, it is still used in the manner which Rorschach himself outlined.

Although other experimenters used ink blots for various research studies, these were concerned primarily with investigating the imagination. Rorschach was actually the first one to use ink blots as a technique for personality diagnosis.

The test itself consists of a series of bilaterally symmetrical ink blots, some black and white and some in color, to which the individual ascribes pictorial representations not inherent in the blot itself. Obviously, because the ink blots do not in reality represent any specific object or objects, there are no wrong or right answers. Each individual looks at the blots and describes what they look like to him. However, in spite of the fact that no evaluation of wrong or right can be applied to the responses, some of the blots have evoked certain fairly common responses. For example, if most people looking at a specific card see, among many other things, at least one configuration in common, and if this card, therefore, consistently elicits a common response like "trees," it would be most significant if an individual were unable to make this perception, particularly after it was pointed out to him. And obviously, an individual who perceives ghosts, witches, hobgoblins, masks, skeletons, etc., to the exclusion of everything else, would certainly differ dramatically from the individual who saw men playing ball, or people on a picnic. Thus an evaluation of the responses in terms of both quality and quantity makes it possible to assess individual personality patterns.

Another widely used projective test of personality is the Thematic

---

[9] P. Lemkau and B. Kronenburg (trans.), H. Rorschach's *Psychodiagnostic: Method and Results of an Experiment in Apperceptual Diagnosis by Means of Interpretation of Random Forms* (New York: Grune & Stratton, 1942).

Apperception Test.[10] This test, somewhat more structured than the Rorschach, presents a series of situational pictures. The subject is requested to invent a story about each picture, telling what events preceded the situation pictured, what is happening in the picture itself, and furthermore, how the story will end. There are thirty pictures in the set, ten of which are used with both men and women, ten with men alone, and ten with women alone. The subject matter of each picture suggests fairly realistic situations; an ambiguous figure leaning against a post, or a woman reading while a man looks over her shoulder. Some of the pictures are more dramatic than others, designed specifically to elicit shock responses, such as a figure lying on a table with a gun and knife in view. The individual who describes this situation as death and destruction is revealing his own problems, as is the individual who describes the same picture as a beneficial operation.

A separate group of cards has also been devised by other researchers for adolescents as well as for children. Whereas the cards designed for adolescents (the Picture Story Test) [11] present pictures of adolescent boys and girls in various situations, the cards presented to children (the Children's Apperception Test) [12] use animal characters. The underlying premise is that young children can identify most readily with animals. Furthermore, it is hypothesized that presenting children with pictures of other children in emotionally charged situations could be excessively traumatic for the young child. It was felt, however, that the child could respond to pictures of animals in emotionally tinged situations and reveal himself without experiencing too much personal stress. These picture situations depict some possible problem aspects in the areas of toilet training, sleep, feeding, and family relationships.

The following examples are actual Rorschach and Children's Apperception Test protocols of two boys, both seven years of age. The

---

[10] H. A. Murray, *Manual for the Thematic Apperception Test* (Cambridge: Harvard University Press, 1943).

[11] P. Symonds, *Adolescent Fantasy* (New York: Columbia University Press, 1949).

[12] L. Bellak and S. Bellak, *Children's Apperception Test* (New York: C. P. S. Co., 1949).

differences between them are quite apparent even to the clinically untrained.

As noted previously, the Rorschach cards consist of unstructured ink blots, some black and white and some in color. The Children's Apperception Test (CAT) is a more structured device consisting of ten pictures which suggest situations and relationships.

TEST RECORD OF NORMAL SEVEN-YEAR-OLD BOY (L.B.)

Rorschach

CARD I: Looks like a pumpkin with eyes cut out—like the kind you have on Halloween.

CARD II: Looks like two elephants holding their trunks together—the red things are circus candy 'cause the elephants are in the circus.

CARD III: Looks like two men with a bow tie between them.

CARD IV: Looks like a thing with two legs—the head is small and the legs are big—I guess it's like—what do you call it?—a big gorilla.

CARD V: Oh, that's a butterfly. It's flying.

CARD VI: That's paint—black paint. Oh, wait, it's a cat. See, it has whiskers like a cat.

CARD VII: Those are doggies.

CARD VIII: Bears climbing up on a mountain.

CARD IX: Those two are animals. Wolves climbing up.

CARD X: Lots of animals all over—here are birds and here are caterpillars and here are dogs.

Children's Apperception Test
[Key: a), description; b), response]

CARD I: a) A picture of chickens sitting at a table eating; the shadow of the mother hen is seen in the background.

b) The three chickens are eating spaghetti. They are finished because their bowls are empty. They ask their mother if they can go out to play and she says, "Yes, but be back in time for dinner." This is lunch —there is a tablecloth.

CARD II: a) A picture of two adult bears tugging at a rope—a baby bear is helping one of them.

b) They are on a picnic playing a game. The baby is with the father— they pull the mother over and they win.

CARD III: a) Picture of a lion sitting in a chair—in one corner is a little mouse.

b) That's a lion who is thinking 'cause he is king. He's making up his mind whether to eat this mouse, but he doesn't 'cause he is king and he's got to be good.

CARD IV: a) Picture of a kangaroo with a baby in her pouch and another kangaroo riding on a bike beside her.

b) This lady—I don't know what you call them—is going shopping—she has milk in the basket—the baby is looking out—the other kid is riding a bike and he wants to get home to watch television.

CARD V: a) Picture of a large double bed and a crib with suggested figures in both of them.

b) This bear is asleep in his crib—he has his toy—he really isn't asleep—just making believe. It's dark in there and he can hear his father snoring.

CARD VI: a) Picture of three animals apparently resting.

b) I don't like this one—everybody is asleep except that one—he's just looking.

CARD VII: a) Picture of a tiger and a monkey.

b) The tiger is running after the monkey—he's hungry—he wants to eat him—he's just ready to bite him when the monkey jumps up in the tree and gets away.

CARD VIII: a) Picture of living room scene with three adult monkeys and one small monkey.

b) That one's a lady and this monkey is talking to the little monkey—must be a lady 'cause there is a flower in her hat.

CARD IX: a) Picture of a rabbit in bed.

b) He's going to sleep, but he's not sleepy. He is listening to his mother and daddy downstairs and he wishes he was watching television too. In a minute he will just go down and watch television.

CARD X: a) Two dogs in a bathroom.

b) They're playing—they are friends and they are playing in the bathroom.

TEST RECORD OF DISTURBED SEVEN-YEAR-OLD BOY (C.R.)

Rorschach

CARD I: Chicken head—looks like on the side.

CARD II: Don't know.

CARD III: Two skeletons with bird heads.

CARD IV: Looks like a dead bear split up in half—you know, cut out.

CARD V: A caterpillar there is crawling into a leaf.

CARD VI: Oh—another one—a dead animal—a cat spread out and split in half.

CARD VII: Here's a little house all crumpled up with rocks falling on it.

CARD VIII: A fire—the animals are running away from it.

And here's two fingers and this is an airplane with water coming out of the wings. Maybe it's putting out the fire and maybe the animals get drowned.

CARD IX: Two witches with green thumbs—here's more water and that's what makes the grass green on the witches' thumbs.

CARD X: A yellow dog with his heart sticking out.

Two rabbit faces and they have one head.

Looks like long skinny worms eating an apple.

A lobster 'cause I see those—and the food the lobster eats is inside him.

I don't see anything else except a little boy.

Children's Apperception Test
[Key: a), description; b), response]

CARD I: a) A picture of chickens sitting at a table eating; the shadow of the mother hen is seen in the background.

b) These chickens are eating chickens (laughs). They're eating their sisters and brothers.

CARD II: a) A picture of two adult bears tugging at a rope—a baby bear is helping one of them.

b) These wolves are playing a game—they're trying to climb a mountain. They get to the top and it's icy and they get stuck for 100 years.

CARD III: a) Picture of a lion sitting in a chair—in one corner is a little mouse.

b) Oh, stupid lion. He was walking in the jungle and he fell down and broke his leg and can't walk any more.

CARD IV: a) Picture of a kangaroo with a baby in her pouch and another kangaroo riding on a bike beside her.

b) Stupid baby, stupid baby, just a stupid baby.

CARD V: a) Picture of a large double bed and a crib with suggested figures in both of them.

b) Ooooh! The mother and father are asleep and the baby climbs out of bed and put his toy in the bed and the mommy thinks the baby turned into a toy. (Has he?) Yes.

CARD VI: a) Picture of three animals apparently resting.

b) This bear is crying 'cause his mother spanked him 'cause he did something bad and he runs away and his mother is sorry he is lost.

CARD VII: a) Picture of a tiger and a monkey.

b) Poor monkey—gets all eaten up.

CARD VIII: a) Picture of living room scene with three adult monkeys and one small monkey.

b) They're talking about him. They say he can't go out to play.

CARD IX: a) Picture of a rabbit in bed.

 b) Sleeping, sleeping, sleeping—always sleeping. He climbs out and the window is open and he runs out.

CARD X: a) Two dogs in a bathroom.

 b) His mommy is spanking him. He threw his toy down the toilet.

While many determinants are used in scoring both the Rorschach and the Children's Apperception Test, it is obvious even by examining only the content aspect of these responses that certain differences can be detected between the two children. On the Rorschach test, the responses of the first child (L.B.) show a pleasant relationship with the environment (circus, candy, Halloween). The second child (C.R.), on the other hand, describes his world in terms of dead animals, crumbling houses, and fires.

Where the first, L.B., was capable of seeing people (Card III), showing that he could identify with the human race, the second, C.R., who saw skeletons with bird heads, could not make this identification. In addition, the bizarre quality of the responses in C.R.'s protocol is found in his flight of ideas and confusion of concepts (Cards VIII, IX, and X).

The same differences are evident on the Children's Apperception Test. L.B.'s satisfactory emotional adjustment is reflected in his stories in which good triumphs over evil (monkey escapes, lion does not eat the mouse, etc.). He indicates concern with the daily activities of his family and feels that he is an integral part of his home environment.

C.R., on the other hand, gives stories replete with aggression. Moreover, his themes indicate destruction and masochism (monkey is eaten, chickens eat sisters and brothers). As in the Rorschach, the bizarre quality of his ideation is also apparent (child becomes toy).

After the complete batteries were evaluated, L.B. was diagnosed as a normal, well-adjusted boy who was integrating his instinctual impulses and was learning to conform to society.

Because of his somewhat tenuous hold on reality, C.R., on the other hand, was diagnosed as severely maladjusted, possibly schizophrenic.

PERSONALITY PROJECTION AS A TEACHING TECHNIQUE

Just as projective tests are used clinically in order to make psychiatric differentiations, so may the concept of projective techniques be put to use in the classroom. The teacher who is capable of using these techniques can develop insights into children's behavior, get a better understanding of their problems, and evaluate their adequacy in coping with these problems. The projective methods that can be used are varied and can be developed in many areas of a school program, particularly through the visual education and language arts programs.

Projective devices may be evolved by the classroom teacher in the form of games. These "games" provide the teacher with additional insights into behavior, and thereby suggest more effective planning for each child in the class. Not only do teachers gain from this program, but children also benefit by being permitted to express feelings and attitudes which ordinarily would have been suppressed. Children are thereby provided with appropriate means for verbally discharging their hostilities and aggressions in socially acceptable ways. The implications of teaching with projective materials are many. A psychologically oriented teacher can become intimately aware of individual children and at the same time enrich the curriculum with opportunities and outlets for spontaneous verbal creativity. Frequently, projective methods offer a first step in establishing rapport. The child, although unaware of the importance and scope of the emotional material he reveals, is making the teacher a part of his past experience on an unconscious level.

It must be emphasized that concern of educators is not with the use of projective tests for diagnosis or therapy in a true clinical sense, and that therefore no standard clinical materials should be used. The techniques that are used in the classroom, while projective in design, are teacher-made. No attempt is made to validate and quantify these classroom materials for standard clinical purposes. They are used informally to study children, particularly those children who appear emotionally disturbed and those whose school adjustment is notably poor. In knowing more about the deviate child, the teacher is better equipped to help him handle problems which are related to school, and in some cases, to extend that help to those peripheral areas which also are disturbing to the child. Classroom use of projective methodology is of particular value, however, to the teacher of the delinquent or emotionally disturbed child in aiding him to understand his attitude toward school, in defining any intolerable pressures related to school, and in evaluating a child's concept of his own particular value in the school constellation. Through the use of projective games, the teacher can become sensitive to those children who are in need of psychiatric help. If some of the children who become disturbed or exhibit antisocial behavior could have been recognized in the classroom through the use of projective methods, then these methods would have been inestimably valuable, from both an educational and a social point of view.

PERSONALITY PROJECTION THROUGH LANGUAGE ARTS

In the language areas, there are several devices that may be used to advantage for personality projection. Modeled after the Kent and Rosanoff Free Association Word Test,[13] a list of words related to school situations, interpersonal relationships, and general school adjustment can be constructed by teachers. This list would include neutral words of no particular emotional tone—such as table, chair, and house—interspersed with such emotionally charged words as school, truant, late, teacher, right, homework, study, principal, friend, and test.

Different types of children respond differently to the stimulus words in line with their own particular needs and tensions. In one classroom, for instance, one boy responded to the word *teacher* with the word *mother;* to *hookey,* the response was *candy;* and to *pencil,* he answered, *suck.* This particular child was in constant need of teacher support. He was dependent, infantile, and inadequate in all social situations. His responses suggest that he was equating the role of the teacher with the role of his mother.

Another boy, who had been in constant difficulty with the law, responded to the same words quite differently. To *teacher,* he responded

---

[13] G. H. Kent and A. J. Rosanoff, "A Study of Association in Insanity", *American Journal of Insanity,* 67 (1910), 37–96, 317–90.

with *character;* to *hookey,* he replied *me;* and to *pencil,* he answered, *knife.* The difference between the two boys, as revealed through this simple projective game, is quite apparent. From just this one game, the teacher could plan differently for each of these children, meeting the needs of each in a more appropriate and realistic manner.

Word association "games" are very versatile. They can be played with one individual or with a group, and can be responded to orally or in writing. Either way, the child would be asked to respond with the first word that comes to his mind as the stimulus word is given. Any very long reaction time or omission should be noted as significant, since hesitancy could be indicative of some emotional blocking. A word association game can be constructed so that it would be completed within a reasonably short period of time. The stimulus words should be selected carefully so that great variety of responses is possible.

A variation of this association projective technique is also possible with a sentence completion "game" consisting, perhaps, of such phrases as:

> When teacher
> My friends
> Report cards
> I'm unhappy in school when
> My school record
> I feel that school
> When my mother comes to school
> Other children in school
> My homework
> When I see the principal it's because
> I had to stay in after school because

When the child is asked to complete these sentences, he is putting down on paper some of his own feelings, thoughts, and attitudes toward school. Sentence completion phrases elicit a great variety of responses which may be indicative of simple personal problems or of severe maladjustment. One boy, age seven, whining and dependent in school, constantly created situations provoking aggression and had to be protected from his classmates. His responses to the sentence completions gave evidence of a much deeper emotional disturbance than could be detected from his classroom behavior alone.

The boy responded to this projective game with these answers:

In school, I like to draw spiders.
My teacher is like an elevator.
I feel that school is on the first floor.
When I see the principal it's because the principal likes octopuses.
My friends in school are children.

The bizarre quality of most of his answers was repeated when he responded to the word association game in the following manner:

house—spider
school—pool
book—look
teacher—house
pencil—star
hookey—moon
table—earth
principal—cobweb

The teacher, on the basis of the unrealistic responses given by this child, became aware of the discrepancy between his overt behavior and his thinking, and recommended intensive psychiatric treatment.

Another classroom device related to word association and sentence completion is story completion. Children love to tell a story as well as listen to one, and even the most disturbed child responds to a story with identification and emotional empathy. Sargent's story completion test of fifteen situations describing a person in conflict [14] can be used as a model by the teacher in constructing story plots for children to finish. The children are asked to embroider the incomplete stories in detail, add as many characters as they choose, and in general to act as author. With this device, the teacher can learn to some extent the strength of environmental pressures upon a particular child, and in addition, gain insights into the developmental thought processes of all

---

[14] H. Sargent, "An Experimental Application of Projective Principles to a Paper and Pencil Personality Test," *Psychological Monographs*, Vol. 57, No. 5 (1944).

children. The following situations, for instance, were given to a group of adolescents:

"A young boy (girl) is studying for a test. His friends call him to go to the movies."

"A boy (girl) is studying for a test. His (her) parents want to go out, but they don't know what to do about leaving him (her) alone at home."

One boy responded to the latter situation with a story which revealed his concept of the role of the parent and his own superficial acceptance of rejection by the parent figures:

"Well, this mother and father, they want to have a good time. They want to go to the saloon, but they don't know what to do with Johnny. It's not nice for a kid to go to a saloon. So his older brother gets a little of this stuff that you put over a guy's face and he goes to sleep. You know what they use in operations, chloroform. So his brother, he thinks he's a big shot, gives the kid the chloroform and off he goes to sleep. Then his mother and father and brother go to the saloon, but he doesn't because it's not nice for kids to go to saloons."

This boy could not accept the parental rejection that he felt, so he compensated for it by explaining that his parents were really interested in his welfare and that his older brother, whom he disliked, was the real villain.

Another story method can also be used which, in some cases, stimulates a freer play of imagination and gives rise to a wider range of phantasy. Teachers may present pictures, perhaps some magazine illustrations, which depict school scenes, but which are vague enough in content to permit a variety of interpretations. For example, as a response to a magazine picture showing a child and a teacher in front of a classroom, in which realistically there was no inference of conflict, the following story was elicited from a fourteen-year-old boy:

"The teacher is scolding the boy. She's telling him he's no good because he stole some money and she's making fun of him in front of the whole class. The boy did steal the money, but he only did it because they needed it at home; his father wasn't working because he's sick. But the teacher doesn't like this kid anyway. She's always picking on him."

A totally different kind of story was elicited from the same picture by another boy, age fifteen:

"Well, this kid won the game for the school team and the teacher is congratulating him. You see, this kid was not allowed on the football team because he was too small and the coach said he could be a substitute only, because he wasn't good enough for the regular team. But during the game on Saturday—this is Monday—they were losing by six points, say forty-five to thirty-nine. And all their team was tired and hurt. And it was the most important game of the season because that game decided whether or not they'd play the championship game. So the coach said, 'Well, I guess we have to send in Lewish.' That's this kid's name. So they sent in Lewish and at the last second, he made a touchdown. He made the final kick, and he won. Well, after all the celebration and everything, this guy is the school hero and the teacher is telling him he could take the day off from school."

It is quite apparent from these stories that the two boys have different problems specific to each of them, and that they responded to the stimulus picture in a manner indicative of those problems. They internalized the material in terms of their own emotional patterns and phantasied an external situation which revealed both their defenses and their conflicts. The first boy was concerned with the poverty of his home, and his story indicated very low self-esteem with definite feelings of rejection by the school authorities.

The story of Lewish as told by Lloyd (the close phonetic similarity of the two names indicates the strength of Lloyd's identification with the fictional character) revealed a boy with an active phantasy life who had great need for being applauded and liked by others. In reality, Lloyd was a big, husky, oversized boy who had not learned to use his height to advantage. He frequently spoke to the other boys of his plans to become a basketball player where his physical size—which he equated with daring and courage—would stand him in good stead. In telling his story, Lloyd was demonstrating his desire to use strength to achieve status in his group.

In order to get a greater variety in storytelling sessions, the same type of material can be presented in an original newspaper chart composed solely of stimulating headlines. This chart is a composite of original and edited headlines set up in the following manner:

FATHER ALWAYS PAYS

EGGS FOR SUPPER

INQUIRIES STARTED
AT DISASTER SCENE

MOM TALKS TO STRANGERS

YOUTH GROUP OPPOSED

PIRATE SHIP SUNK

COTTON CANDY HAIR

HIS WORLD WAS MADE OF RUBBER

HE DIES OFTEN,
BUT HE NEVER
HAS BEEN A
CORPSE

Using this chart, children choose their own headlines and write a story about them. The choice of the headline is the child's, not the teacher's, which in itself is projective in nature. The added story, of course, gives further information about the child. For instance, a book review headed, "His World Was Made of Rubber," used the title of the biography of Harvey Firestone. Using this headline as the stimulus, a very controlled boy with good defenses gave the following story:

"This man was hypnotized and he said he went to a different planet. He only said he went to a planet, but he didn't go. It was all his imagination. He was dreaming. It was in his imagination, but at the end it was true. His house was made of rubber and when the bombs from the planet fell down, his rubber house just could bend over and the bombs couldn't hit it and it was saved. Then he came back to earth. It just goes to show, at the end it happens and it comes true. Like when the world was round, everybody said it was square, but they found out it was round. Well, they could find out it's good when a house is made of rubber."

This story proved to be particularly interesting because this boy, who had adequate control of his impulses, would sometimes lose his control and act in a very aggressive bizarre manner. Evidences of his breaks with reality in behavior were reinforced in this story, which starts as fiction, vacillates between phantasy and reality, but which actually he ends up believing.

Children like telling stories whether a visual or an oral stimulus is used. Playing a little round-robin talking game is another way of obtaining projected material. By going around the class in turn, each pupil can be asked to say the first thing that comes to his mind. The following remarks are indicative of the problems, thoughts, and feelings expressing the concerns of a group of emotionally disturbed children:

JOHN, age 9: I like to eat. I like to eat naked peanut butter, I mean without bread.

SEON, age 9: One thing I don't like about my mother. She likes to love me too much. I don't like too much love. It gives me the creeps.

FRANK, age 10: Once upon a time this little boy's father lived in the jungle. There were big dinosaurs, crocodiles, and all kinds of giants. The boy went out. He got eaten up. That's the end. Oh yes, there was an earthquake.

ETHAN, age 10: Nothing.

RUSSELL, age 10: School, I hate it.

DAVID, age 13: The teacher says he wants to be a nice small butterfly so he can sneak through screens. He wants to be a lot of pretty colors. Why would a teacher want to be a butterfly?

From the children's own expressions, the teacher saw that Seon, for instance, rather than describing an actuality, was reflecting an intense wish for love. It is interesting, however, that not having experienced such love, he rationalized the situation by denying his need for it. The problems of the other children also stand revealed. John gives evidence of needing affection in the form of food, and he equates being fed with being loved. Frank was concerned with aggression and explosive destruction. Russell, also an aggressive child, merely expressed his negative feeling toward school, showing he could control this feeling. David was unrealistic, perhaps voicing a particular phantasy at this moment.

Ethan, however, was too inhibited, fearful, or cautious to permit himself any kind of expression. He was not pressured into further communication, for at this time pressure would have led to resistance and antagonism. Several days later, however, Ethan was comfortable enough to give expression to his concerns. From his written story, it is easy to see why he might block at expressing it orally. He was so caught up with aggressive feelings toward his mother that he was unable to verbalize openly. He was afraid to give free expression to his impulses and afraid his emotions would be overpowering. The only way he could control his feelings, the first time he was approached, was to suppress them. Subsequently he wrote the following:

"Mr. X. is a bird-person-magician. Mr. X. has wings of a bird, the legs of a person, and can be invisible like a magician. Mr. X. lives in Fairy Land. Mr. X.'s only enemy was the Black Fairy of Turtlesville.

"Right now, Mr. X. is locked in the tower of the Black Fairy. Well, when it was about lunch time, the Black Fairy would come up to the room where Mr. X. was locked and give him bread and water. Well, it was about lunch time and the Black Fairy opened the door. Well, where was he? He was invisible. When the Black Fairy looked for him he made himself visible, kicked her and flew out the door. She got up flying after him. Well, Mr. X. flew to Arizona, U.S.A.

"Mr. X. flew over an Indian Village and landed in an empty tent. When the Black Fairy landed she landed in the middle of the village. All of a sudden the Indians pounced on her. They thought she was an evil spirit. They tied her to the stake and burned her. That's the way most bad people end."

The Black Fairy probably represents the mother figure, or perhaps a fusion of both parents. Mr. X. appears to be symbolic of the child himself. Originally his concept of the mother figure, or mother-father fusion image, however, seemed to be so threatening that to handle these feelings he had to resort to suppression. It is interesting, however, that in the written story the mother-father figure is killed off. It is probably an expression of Ethan's unconscious death wishes against his parents. It is also possible that this unconscious death wish was the feeling with which the child was struggling at the moment that this particular projective game was played.

Another particularly evocative projective game may be called the "Six Wishes." In this game, the child is asked the following questions:

1. If you could have any kind of world to live in, what kind of world would it be?
2. If you could have any kind of family, what kind of family would it be? Who would be in it?
3. If you could have anybody in the world for a friend, who would it be? (Why?)
4. If you could be anything or anybody you wanted, what or who would you be? (Why?)
5. If there was one thing you could do all day long without stopping, what would it be? (Why?)
6. If you could pick your dream at night, what would it be?

It is interesting to compare the answers of a seriously disturbed child with those of a normal, well-adjusted child. The following case history is that of a disturbed boy.

Charles is a twelve-year-old white Catholic boy who lives with his mother and father and six siblings. He has three brothers, ages nine, six and four; and three sisters, ages eight and two—the latter, a pair of twins. His father is a mechanic who makes a good living and the home is physically adequate.

Although both his mother and father are known to be very punitive, subjecting the children to frequent beatings, Charles says he loves them. Charles would like to move to another neighborhood because he feels that the neighborhood is a source of difficulty for him. He constantly gets into fights with other children because, as he says, "Everybody picks on me, even the grocery man. They don't like me, nobody does."

Charles is in the sixth grade. He obtained an IQ of 109 on the Stanford-Binet Scale, Form L. He is retarded in both arithmetic and reading. His arithmetic grade on the Woody-McCall Arithmetic Test was 3.6. On the Gilmore Reading Test, Form A, he obtained a reading grade of 2.9.

Charles' teacher described him in the following terms: "Charles is a very pale child who stammers and never mixes with the other children in my class. He always has a faraway look and is always getting hurt. He seems to be accident prone and actually invites abuse from the other boys. He is a frequent truant, and at these times, I understand, he does not come to school because he runs away from home. He even stays away all night."

Charles' six wishes consisted of the following answers:

1. If you could have any kind of world to live in, what kind of world would it be?

"I would have all the crooks in jail. No one could curse without being fined $10.00. There would be free movies every night and I would build extra theaters. Everyone in the world would have a five-room apartment. There would be playgrounds on every street and lots more swimming pools. I would send men out to kill all the germs so they can't give us disease.

"Everyone would have to go swimming and build houses every day—I'd make that a law. People should give plays for other people—then we could all stay up till three in the morning. I'd like that, I've been up all night. Anyone who didn't do as I said—they'd be put to death—no, not that— that's too much—they won't get food for three weeks—that way I'll still have workers and I'd be a real boss. No one could escape—if they tried, they'd get seven years in jail—if they try again, then life.

"I'd have rubber streets and rubber houses so that the streets could move apart and the houses could sway and bend over a bit and then bombs couldn't hit them.

"I'd have thirty space ships in case we are attacked, and we could charge them with power guns, power hoses, jet suits and gravity pullers. I'd have 100 submarines and if an enemy tried to charge us I'd have 50,000 airplanes, 2000 gun fields and two million speedboats.

"England would get all the tobacco fields.

"Germany would have very nice houses.

"Taxes would be $2.00 a year for each person in the world. Money would be made every week—one million dollars each week. I'd have bathing shows, pond races—where ducks race—everything free."

2. If you could have any kind of family, what kind of family would it be? Who would be in it?

"I would take my mother, father, sister, and the twins. Billy, Jimmy, and John, my brothers, can stay behind—maybe in Japan. My mother will have a new dress every day—my father a new suit every day, and I'd have the biggest diamond in the world—the most expensive—an emerald one. I'd wear a new tie every year. It would take me ten weeks to save up for a new tie at one million dollars a week. I'd have a pretty wife—blond hair, blue eyes, red cheeks, rosy lips, and nice build."

3. If you could have anybody in the world for a friend, who would it be?

"I would have all the people in the world for friends and they would have to do what I wanted, or I'd put them in jail."

4. If you could be anything or anybody you wanted, what or who would you be?

"I'd be the owner of this world—I wouldn't have a job. I'd just swim and have fun and take it easy like President Eisenhower does—not even sign papers—I'd have a signing machine."

5. If there was one thing you could do all day long without stopping, what would it be?

"I'd swim all day long—I dive into the water—I bet you walk in—but I can swim, I'm a water bug. I can swim 100 feet underwater—I did it all the time—I'm a real water bug."

6. If you could pick your dream at night, what would it be?

"I'd dream about guns—shooting down those lousy crooks. I'd have my special submarine and I wouldn't even be tired in the morning. The special submarine is really me. I told you I'm a water bug. I'd be a submarine. I'm always a submarine at night."

Many of Charles' problems were reflected in his wishes. He was certainly unrealistic and bizarre, giving evidence of extreme aggressive phantasy and seeing himself as an authoritarian, destructive figure. His concern with space, numbers, and time was almost obsessive, as if he were trying to identify himself in time and space. His feelings of inadequacy seemed to be compensated by power-driven activities.

Psychiatric evaluation revealed much the same mechanisms. Charles was described by the psychologist as "trying to maintain his own status through primitive phantasy and inadequate impulsive acting-out behavior. His essential behavior appears to be his inability to recognize his own value as a human being and an inability to maintain an adequate ego structure. Because of his inability to find himself in time and space, his lack of self-concept, and subsequent breaks with reality, the diagnosis of schizophrenia must be made."

The teacher, of course, merely on the basis of this game, would not have made a definite diagnosis of schizophrenia, although a guess could have been hazarded that this child was psychotic. Certainly, his gross disturbance would not have gone undetected even from just his wish responses.

Charles was very verbal in his responses. He enjoyed the game and relished the idea of talking to the class. In fact, his flight of ideas were almost compulsive in nature, and he seemed unable to stop talking even when he was told to give another child a chance.

All children do not respond as readily as Charles did. It is probably correct to say that normal children are slightly hesitant in revealing themselves before a class, even when they know it is a game. Usually, there is more embarrassment, attributable to better defense mechanisms, and the child appears reluctant to talk about himself in front of others. Most of the time, however, this reluctance is overcome as soon as the child accepts the game as fun.

Susan, a normal, well-adjusted youngster, was at first hesitant about joining this game. However, when she did participate she seemed to enjoy it. The following record was given by Susan and is as indicative of her personality as Charles' record was reflective of his:

1. If you could have any kind of world to live in, what kind of world would it be?

"Oh, it would have nice houses with nice families in them. And all the children would go to school and all the men would work and everybody would have a car and washing machines and things like that."

2. If you could have any kind of family, what kind of family would it be? Who would be in it?

"My mother and father and me and my baby sister. Well, sometimes (at this point she laughed), well, sometimes, she takes my crayons and messes my toys and I wish—well, she's only two. My mother says she has to learn things. I guess she will."

3. If you could have anybody in the world for a friend, who would it be?

"Roberta is my best friend. She lives on my block and we go to school together every day, and we play every afternoon. She's my best friend 'cause I like her and she likes me."

4. If you could be anything or anybody you wanted, what or who would you be?

(Laughed) "Myself. I'd be myself. (After much urging by the teacher, she continued.) Well, maybe I'd like to be a nurse in a hospital. My daddy is a doctor and he says nurses are very, very important."

5. If there was one thing you could do all day long without stopping, what would it be?

"I don't know. I like to go ice skating. Maybe I'd like to ice skate all day, that is, if I didn't get tired. Nothing else."

6. If you could pick your dream at night, what would it be?

"Oh, I like to read about princesses and fairy tales and things like that. Maybe I'd like to dream about that—you know—like a story I never have, but I'd like to."

Susan is a nine-year-old child in the fourth grade. On the Revised Stanford-Binet Scale, Form L, she obtained an IQ of 123, which places her in the superior range of the population. She is the oldest of three children, two girls, five and two respectively. The family unit appears to be a happy one.

On achievement tests, Susan achieved a reading grade of 4.7 on the Gilmore Reading Test, Form A; an arithmetic grade of 4.4 on the Woody-McCall Arithmetic Test. She is, therefore, working on grade level. She probably, however, has the capacity to function slightly higher.

The teacher describes Susan as "a happy, well-adjusted child. Her work is good. She has many friends and seems to like school. The only difficulty is, sometimes she chatters too much, and she's inclined to be bossy. But these are no problems, really."

Susan's answers reflect her basically happy frame of mind. She is content with the world as she finds it. On the question of who or what she would like to be, she answers that she wants to be herself, or possibly a nurse when she grows up. Charles, on the other hand, didn't wait to grow up. He impulsively and immediately wanted to be "boss of the world." Whereas Susan realistically keeps her own friend when asked with whom she would like to be friends, Charles replies that everybody in the world will be his friend. Again, Susan is demonstrating her satisfaction with the world as she finds it, and with her own role in it, while Charles is searching for something that cannot possibly exist.

Although Susan expresses some dissatisfaction with her baby sister, at the same time she was willing to cope with the problem. She will wait for the baby "to learn" to do things as her mother tells her she must. Charles, however, could never show any such sympathetic tolerance. He must rule, abuse, and destroy in an attempt to prove his own value.

A psychological interview revealed much of the same findings concerning Susan that the "Six Wishes" game revealed. The psychologist's evaluation stated briefly that Susan "appears to be functioning adequately within her environment. Although she occasionally reverts to immature behavior and some impulsive acting-out, she gives every indication of being a 'normal,' well-adjusted child."

A comparison of the six wishes of both Susan and Charles quickly indicates that each child has revealed the core of his own personality patterning. Such a revelation, moreover, reflects not only the forces of the environment in which each child lives, but also indicates the way in which each child views his own role in that environment.

PERSONALITY PROJECTION THROUGH VISUAL AIDS

Teachers today are familiar with visual-aid materials and methods. Filmstrips, silent films, and sound films play a part in presenting new material or in reviewing previously taught material. This purpose of visual aids is very well known and widely used. Less widely used, however, are visual aids as tools for personality projection.

Children respond projectively to any little segment of a film which has some special personal meaning even though that portion may be an insignificant part of the entire film. Films used to elicit projective material may be either instructional or entertaining, concerned with objects and symbols or with real life situations and real people. Identification and emotional release can be attained from any film subject. Troubled children, particularly, react with intensity and absorption, selecting the material in a film which is meaningful to them personally.

The teacher can almost never determine in advance the kind of reaction a film will evoke. The film presented is chosen first for the teaching possibilities it offers and second for the emotional release it may give the children. Particular films, however, act as a better stimulus than others in provoking projection.

A projective visual-aid program is equally effective whether discussion follows immediately after the film, or concurrently, as might be done with filmstrips. Discussion can be either on a personal basis between the pupil and teacher alone, or on a group basis with the class participating. In group discussions, the teacher can observe interpersonal relations within the group, as well as the personal reactions to the film.

The following discussion by a group of disturbed youngsters, ages nine and ten, is representative of the type of reaction that is frequently found among such troubled children. The discussion was held as the filmstrip "Jack and the Beanstalk" was being presented. One particular frame, depicting Jack climbing the stalk, seemed to be a rather innocuous one, but it came immediately after a frame in which Jack had been scolded by his mother for having brought home the magic bean. The spontaneous conversation of a group of disturbed children in relation to the frame on climbing follows:

MICHAEL: Stupid Jack, he'll get hurt climbing like that.
JUAN: You think he's soft like you, eh? He wants to be rich so his mother will like him. His mother likes him, but she'll like him better when he's rich.
ALFRED: Nobody likes him, nobody does, 'cause he's bad.
MICHAEL: He'll get hurt.
ALFRED: Like when I beat you up.
VIRGINIA: His mother won't care. She wants him to get hurt. She would like to get rid of him, that's what.
ALFRED: Yeah, he's bad.
JUAN: Well, I don't know about that.

Later, with the presentation of a frame wherein Jack is seen hiding from the giant and seeking refuge in the stove, Michael's concern about his physical safety, as well as Virginia's extreme feeling of rejection were clearly defined. Juan's apparent ambivalent attitude to his mother was once more expressed and Alfred showed his lack of self-esteem and his tendency toward aggression. It was also evident that Michael is Alfred's particular target of aggression. The following is part of the verbatim conversation:

JUAN: If he doesn't get out, his mother will worry.
VIRGINIA: She's an old hag. She won't worry. She wants him burned.
JUAN: Maybe she does, but only when he's bad.
ALFRED: He's a no-good guy. I don't like him either.
VIRGINIA: Neither do I.
MICHAEL: I like him.
ALFRED: Who cares what you like?
VIRGINIA: Yeah, who cares?

It is interesting to note that in "Jack and the Beanstalk" the role of the mother is an exceedingly small one. She appears in only three frames. Still, these children reacted to the mother as though she were the core of the story, and the discussion centered upon her. While discussion can start spontaneously, only adroit questioning can maintain it for any length of time so that the teacher can explore individual reactions.

It is readily observable that a teacher can gain many valuable insights into the behavior of the children through reported conversations such as those presented. With this particular group, additional insight was obtained a week later when the teacher presented a sixteen-millimeter sound film on the butterfly and its development from the caterpillar. At the completion of the film, the children were extremely excited about the wonderful change the caterpillar had achieved by becoming a butterfly. The discussion that follows indicates that the very same concerns that were apparent in the discussion of "Jack and the Beanstalk" are revealed in relation to the caterpillar and the butterfly:

VIRGINIA: I would like to change like that. Only my mother will be a fairy princess, not a stepmother.
MICHAEL: I'll be Mighty Mouse so nobody will hurt me, or maybe a porcupine so I can stick people.
ALFRED: I'll be Superman and kill all the criminals.
JUAN: I won't be anybody but myself, just Juan. But I'd like to be rich. Maybe a king, and everybody will have to do what I tell them—even my mother.
VIRGINIA: But stepmothers are all right if they are fairy princesses, too.
ALFRED: That's stupid.

MICHAEL: That's stupid.
ALFRED: (To Michael) You shut up.

The teacher can use visual aids as a key to personality projection not only with young children, but also with older children and adolescents. It is not unusual for adolescent boys and girls to be interested in fairy tales which have an emotional impact, even though they may evidence superficial disdain for such infantile fare.

For instance, the filmstrip of "Cinderella" held the attention of a group of adolescents throughout the showing. The subsequent discussion became quite heated, particularly when it centered upon the cruelty of the siblings and the stepmother. It was then relatively easy to discover which of the children came from homes where they seemed to be less favored than other members of the family. More specifically, the teacher discovered which figures in the family constellation engendered resentment simply by noting the character of greatest concern—the cruel stepmother, the favored siblings, or perhaps the force of an unknown good, centered in the fairy godmother who was a benefactor only until midnight. It was significant that throughout this film one particular girl identified the fairy godmother with her own inconsistent mother, who gave favors only to rescind them later.

This particular filmstrip offered insights into the difficulties of several children who stood out as school problems, helping the teacher grow in understanding of each child's overt behavior. The older girl who resented the fairy godmother, for instance, was continually rebelling against the adult authority of the teacher. It was, in fact, not the teacher who was the core of her problem, but rather her attitude toward the authority in her home and her mother, whose affection was never seen as certain.

The value of projection with visual aids is enhanced by permitting the teacher to discover a personal problem even though this problem may not be related specifically to school. Louis, a case in point, reacted as follows to a filmstrip:

Louis, age 14, seemed to like school and to get along well. The teacher noted that Louis never participated in a group unless he was specifically

invited to do so. If no one suggested that he become part of a group, he
would not do so of his own accord. One day a filmstrip was presented which
was part of the science lesson. The class had just set up an aquarium and
were watching a filmstrip on aquariums. As a minor part of the film, there
was a slight explanation of the life cycle of a fish, beginning with the egg-
laying process. During this presentation and the discussion that ensued
with each frame as it was presented, Louis broke out spontaneously with,
"Look at that old lady fish! She goes and leaves her babies like that and
waits for somebody to come along and take care of them. It's all wrong!"

His diatribe was just a brief explosion and most of the children in
the class seemed not to notice his outburst. After the film was completed, however, the teacher guided the discussion to methods other
fish and animals used in caring for their young. Was it all wrong, as
Louis had said, for a mother to leave her eggs? During this session
Louis expressed his resentment openly, and the teacher learned a
great deal about him and the extreme rejection he felt he was suffering
from his own mother. The teacher also realized that perhaps Louis'
behavior—his unaggressive participation and his extreme reticence
when invited to join a group—stemmed from this feeling of maternal
rejection. Louis withdrew and conformed perhaps because he could not
face the possibility of being rejected in the classroom as he felt he was
at home.

With this additional understanding, the teacher was able to plan for
specific successful activities for Louis which would enhance his sense
of security and help him build a better concept of himself by providing
opportunities to be constantly accepted by both the teacher and his own
peers. Without the aid of this film, the teacher might possibly never
have discovered Louis' feelings of rejection. As it was, through the use
of this film, Louis' problem was easily discernible and steps were taken
to help him adjust to his own situation.

Summary

Clinical psychologists use many projective devices for diagnostic purposes. However, projective devices may be used not only by the clini-
cian, but also by the classroom teacher who is interested not in
diagnosing pathologies, but in children. The teacher wants to know

each child in the room very well, and some of the children especially well. Some such insights may be obtained through the projective use of the visual-aid program and the language arts curriculum.

The teacher, like the psychologist, wants to study and know the emotional personality of each child. The use the teacher makes of this information differs from that of the psychologist, but the teacher recognizes a sound pedagogical and psychological principle which states that meeting a child's educational needs must include meeting his emotional needs.

Information which is necessary for something more than a casual understanding of the child is not always available on a record card, and indeed it should not be made part of a permanent public record. Such information, moreover, cannot always be obtained just by observation or interview. Although the teacher makes use of all these procedures and many more, projection as a separate educational tool cannot be overestimated as a valuable technique in reaching a better understanding of children.

Chapter X

The Creative Arts

The creative arts program for the emotionally disturbed child is conceived as basic to education for adjustment. It has as its prime objective not the teaching of skill, but rather the natural unfolding of creative potential, which helps channelize undesirable impulses into constructive activities. The creative arts are unique in that in this area alone every child is an expert—he need be only himself to be successful and productive. Here alone the teacher says, "Don't do it my way, do it your way. I am interested in you and what you have to say—and I like the way you say it." Confidence in oneself is inherent in making school a satisfying experience for the maladjusted child, permitting the release of inner tensions and the expression of individuality in a socially acceptable manner. Creative artistic expression, whether in painting, drawing, sculpture, music, or dancing has its emphasis in the word "creative," and uses the tools of the arts for stimulating the spontaneous expressions of each individual according to his own measure. It provides the pattern for emotional maturation and personality development, offering therapeutic restoration as well as insights into psychological processes. Thus, opportunities for creative artistic expression are clearly related not only to eventual improvement in academic skills, but even more basically, to resolving emotional conflicts and redirecting undesirable behavior.

Achievement in art depends primarily upon the courage to be oneself, and the knowledge that one can be oneself successfully. Here learning is based not on step-by-step sequentially planned instruction, but on unlimited freedom of self-expression for each individual, according to his own needs and at his own level of functioning. In academic areas the teacher is the expert imparting knowledge and setting standards. In art the child is the expert. Two little red lines can be a horse, a birthday cake, or even Superman. As the artist sees them, so they are. His unique way of thinking, feeling, and perceiving are valued infinitely above his ability to acquire knowledge and skills. He can ignore reality and disregard reason. His themes can be bizarre, his colors inappropriate, and his choice of media incongruous by adult standards. But if they are his own direct expressions, the child has succeeded, not only on his own terms, but in relation to the demands of the school structure. He is free to paint a green man hanging on a red tree or a red moon grinning in a black sky; he can draw a cow with three heads, or a house running away from a fire. His well-pounded lump of clay can turn into a dinosaur or a dead mouse. Whatever he has to say is interesting and worth serious attention.

For praise and approval he need be only himself, and this no one can teach him. Art can be his best friend, helping him pictorialize his problems when words or actions are either inadequate or inadmissible. In practical terms, this means that a child's drawing of a boy kicking his dog relieves pent-up aggressive impulses, and serves, to a large extent, the same function as actual kicking. Such nonverbal communications are welcomed by the teacher as a means of helping the child express his complaints without hurting himself or others. With the teacher's approval, he discovers that he need not be ashamed of his thoughts, emotions, and phantasies. He is constantly encouraged to externalize his inner tensions and resolve his emotional conflicts through graphic expression. The resultant cathartic release gives the disturbed child a feeling of inner completeness. By bringing unconscious problems into conscious organization, he experiences a relaxation and a reduction of anxiety. He displaces the negative behavior generated by frustrating situations and compensates for his lack of academic achievement in a socially acceptable way. This process is therapeutic.

In these terms, art as a therapeutic experience provides the disturbed child with goals which are within his reach. He begins to understand the universality of human emotions—that fear, anger, tenderness, pity, love, and hate are acceptable, basic normal feelings. Particularly, he is learning that feelings are neither good nor bad of themselves, but only in the form they take for expression. When the need for expressing these emotions is satisfied better by constructive creative artistic experiences than by the former undesirable behavior, the disturbed child is being restored. He is making a positive emotional investment and enhancing his self-esteem. He is setting the stage for emotional maturation, social re-education, and academic remediation.

The teacher's role in this art education process is both easy and difficult. No teacher need shy away from planning art activities because of a lack of talent or training. Art education, from this point of view, is seen not as *teaching* art, but rather as fostering creative self-expression—employing the versatile tools of art for stimulating spontaneity and individuality. This approach, however, does not imply a hands-off, laissez-faire policy. While creativity in artistic expression cannot be taught, it certainly can be encouraged. The teacher plays a very active role by providing materials and by motivating, cajoling, and enticing the child into feeling that art is fun—that art is a vitalizing, freedom-loving, confidence-building activity. The rigid, compulsive child can delicately approach finger paints by using only the tip of one finger for as long as he feels the need for this restriction. The aggressive child may express his hostility by repeatedly painting scenes of violence, while the shy, withdrawn child may find release in perseverative repetitions of a somber, dark design.

Jose, for example, a withdrawn, unsmiling Puerto Rican boy of ten, repeatedly painted the top half of a sheet of paper red and the bottom half black. He literally reiterated this same design over thirty times. At every opportunity the teacher would say, "Tell me about it." Each time the child answered, "Country." The teacher tried to stimulate him by placing new, brightly colored paints in front of his darker ones, and by providing him with both crayons and chalk. But Jose clung tenaciously to his one somber theme. Thirty-three times the teacher thanked him for his picture, patted him on the head, and praised his efforts by displaying his work—and thirty-three times he gave no evidence of being aware of her presence. The thirty-fourth time, however, a subtle change took place—the red was considerably lighter and the black was blended with green.

Gradually, the black was replaced with a bright green and the red with a lovely pale blue. While the basic pattern remained the same, lo and behold! one day the green gave birth to a tree covered with very distinct little red fruits and a fat sun appeared in the light blue sky. Simultaneously, a small, melancholy, withdrawn boy managed to smile at the teacher.

As a result of this cathartic experience, Jose was able, somehow, to come to terms with his problem. An examination of his case history revealed that his father had died a few weeks before, and his mother had sent him from Puerto Rico to New York to live with relatives. His distress at this unhappy turn of events gave rise to behavioral symptoms—he ran away from his new home several times, and finally, when he was caught in an attempt to stow away on a tramp steamer, he came to the attention of the courts. Here he was recognized as a problem, and placed in a psychiatric hospital.

His art expressions were clearly a reflection of the bleak, barren, isolated feelings he was experiencing. Alone, far from home, and feeling rejected by those he loved, he could not mobilize his resources to meet his inner desperation. Since depression, withdrawal, and a language barrier combined to prevent easy communication, pictorial representations were his most natural means of expression. The therapeutic environment, coupled with a sympathetic, accepting teacher, permitted him to objectify his feelings and eventually work through his depression. He could now channel his energies toward facing life with a bit more courage and confidence. Little by little his behavior changed— he began to participate in group activities, learned to speak English, and after four months, was returned to his relatives. He entered a regular school in New York City and has been making excellent progress.

This boy is not an isolated case. His story, with infinite variations, has been repeated many times. Howard was a thirteen-year-old, violently aggressive boy who approached the therapeutic art experience by promptly smashing six new full pint jars of paint. He extended himself over and over again to test the limits of the teacher's patience. When he discovered that the teacher refused to reject him, meeting each assault with renewed attempts to interest him in painting, he finally accepted the challenge. He could not believe, however, that he as an individual was accepted, in spite of the fact that his behavior was clearly unacceptable. His first production was a bloody mess of red paint—a nude with a dagger in her chest. With obvious belligerence he presented his picture to the teacher. Once more he was testing the limits. When the teacher said he had done well with a most difficult subject and she was proud of his work, he was stunned. It was almost pathetic to hear him say, "Hey, you know teach, this is the first time a teacher said I done anything good!"

The turning point in Howard's adjustment had come. His art work remained violent in content, but his bold primary colors were now interspersed with muted pastel shades. He began, also, to limit his conceptions so that his drawing or painting could be contained on the paper instead of spilling off in all directions. He experimented with clay, with wood carving, textures, and collages. Although progress was neither smooth nor consecutive, his temper tantrums diminished, his hostility dissipated, and his overt behavior improved considerably. Howard really reached a new level of emotional maturity, however, when one day he admitted to the teacher that he could not read, and moreover, that now he wanted to learn how.

Persistent themes may be as superficially innocuous as Jose's landscape, or as sadistic and aggressive in content as Howard's drawings. Jack, age sixteen, whose conflict centered on his aggressive drives, gave expression to these drives in hundreds of weird, bizarre themes. He drew many two-headed figures, and in explaining his drawings, verbalized his own emotional ambivalence. One head wanted to kill, while the other asked for help to stop the first from committing murder. Jack was clearly asking to be saved from himself. The duality of impulses, so often associated with schizophrenia, expressed the conflict between internal unconscious drives and the conscious values of reality.

As Jack improved, while his themes were still bizarre, he managed to give them some overt semblance of acceptability. This same boy found satisfaction in other creative expressions. He wrote an autobiography, learned to play the piano, began to write little songs, and started a large record collection. With all these emotional outlets, he managed to function with some adequacy. His acceptable behavior increased and his interests were used in planning a vocational goal. He later managed to obtain admission to a piano-tuning school, and shows promise of becoming a productive member of society.

The therapeutic value of these free expressions can be fully realized only if the teacher understands their function and is not inclined to moralize about the content. These revelations can also be used to provide the teacher with insights into individual problems. In a drawing of war (a frequent theme for boys) instead of using large, bold strokes, Juan confined himself to tiny lines drawn mostly with the aid of a ruler. Although Juan's theme was aggressive, it was apparent from the small size of the figures and the heavy lines which had been repeatedly reinforced, that he was holding back his aggressive impulses. Dark, ominous clouds, also, were restrained by the use of restrictive, rigid lines. There was no spontaneity in the picture, and the stiff clean pencil lines reflected Juan's repression. This child was clearly trying to inhibit and control his own impulses as well as the environment itself. This was reflected by his use of rigid lines to contain the figures in his drawing.

Repressive elements also find expression in the size of the drawing. Unhappy, withdrawn children very often draw to a minute scale. Their landscapes may be rigidly constructed with small trees, houses, and flowers. People, if any are represented, are tiny. Because these children are holding back their emotions, they do not like to use media which demand bold strokes and spontaneity. Repressed children often draw rather than paint, and prefer pencil and ruler rather than crayons. Children who are emotionally constricted often resort to geometric designs to the exclusion of any representational expression. Such attempts to control the environment are most often seen in neurotic children who in their compulsive mechanisms attempt to circumscribe the world about them. In Joseph's pencil drawing of different kinds of food, each type of food in turn suggested another, and in an anxiety-driven, compulsive manner he attempted to put on paper many kinds of food. It was not enough to draw them, however, he also had to identify them. Letters, written in English and Greek, were used interchangeably. (Joseph was from Greece and had been in the United States only a few years.) The food theme reflected Joseph's feelings of oral deprivation and his search for a mother figure who would give him warmth and a loving relationship, a need that food represented to him. Thus he expressed his regression with a theme that indicated his infantile level of development.

Since drawing is reflective of emotional life and developmental level, it has been used extensively by psychologists in the analysis of personality. Drawings of the human figure, in particular, have been valuable in both the analysis of personality and the evaluation of intelligence. Florence Goodenough devised a rating scale by which a figure drawing made by a child can be analyzed and scored so that a mental age and an IQ may be obtained.[1] Karen Machover, using the same figure, devised a means of analyzing the drawing from a psychological point of view.[2] Without elaboration, the child is merely told to draw a whole person. Usually, boys draw the male figure, while girls draw the female figure.

Many children, particularly adolescents, object to drawing a human figure because they do not draw well. The adolescent who does not draw freely is often embarrassed about his inadequacy in drawing and may have to be coerced a bit. Eventually, however, most adolescents will comply, particularly when the request is made during a psychological testing session. When persons are obstinate and refuse to draw at all, they are giving evidence of severe constriction and rigidity. They will not draw because they fear that their drawings will be too revealing of themselves. In any case, these persons are denying the situation and withdrawing from it.

---

[1] F. L. Goodenough, *Measurement of Intelligence by Drawing* (New York: World Book Co., 1926).

[2] K. Machover, *Personality Projection in the Drawing of the Human Figure* (Springfield, Ill.: Charles C. Thomas, Publisher, 1949).

Children generally draw figures from a full-face view. With sophistication, however, particularly in adolescence, the profile view is attempted. If a profile or back view is elicited when a child is expressly asked to draw a front view, he may be expressing avoidance or withdrawal tendencies. In other words, he may be refusing to "face up" to things.

In drawing human figures, most children will start with the head, then draw the trunk, body, arms, and so forth. Schizophrenic children, however, without any direction other than "draw a whole person," often start by drawing a hand or a foot first. Frequently, these same children start an animal by drawing the hooves first. Occasionally this drawing of the extremities is submitted by the child as the whole person. In some cases, the child may even trace his own hand and call it his body. Such children are apparently not capable of recognizing that important parts of the figure are omitted. This is certainly a bizarre fact, particularly when one considers that while normal young children will offer a head as a complete person, they would never give an isolated trunk, neck, leg, or arm as a representation of a complete person. Schizophrenic children, however, frequently draw such body extremities.

It might be hypothesized that this kind of drawing is so prevalent because the act of picking up the pencil or crayon to draw causes the child to become aware of his own hand. In addition, he becomes aware of the lack of muscle tone, a condition characteristic of schizophrenic children. This small act—clutching a pencil—which is normally a weak muscular feat, is a strong physical change in the schizophrenic's hand-body sense, and directs attention to this organ abruptly, forcing concentration upon the hand. The child then proceeds to center his activity on the part of his body of which he is most aware at the moment; he draws the hand. It is also possible that in drawing the hand, the schizophrenic child is attempting to establish and maintain his own ego. He uses his hand to reach out into the environment, to try to find his own place within a reality that he does not fully comprehend. By drawing the hand, he is attempting to establish his own body boundaries.

In a recent experiment, the authors asked children to draw a good person and a bad person. This experiment was not limited to disturbed children alone, but included hundreds of children attending the regular grades in the public schools. Each child was presented with paper and asked to draw two persons, a bad person and a good person. No further instructions were given. A comparison of the drawings of both groups of children, disturbed and nondisturbed, gave some interesting results that are worth noting. Specifically, it may be stated that both groups of children showed, in their concepts of good and bad, certain common characteristics. These characteristics are summarized as follows:

1. The good person was most often drawn first. Possibly this was so because the figure was less traumatic and the concept less threatening.
2. The bad person was drawn in the act of doing something with his hands. Older children made the picture situational—a man was holding up a bank, or riding away from a robbery on a horse. Some figures had just set fire to a house. Others had already been caught and were placed behind bars.
3. The bad figure generally had no neck at all, or a very much smaller neck than the figure of the good person. Machover [3] considers that the neck probably represents the organ of control. It is that part of the body which separates the impulses associated with the body and trunk from the intellectual controls represented by the head. Thus, a short neck, or no neck at all, may represent the lack of control which the child associates with badness. A good person has a longer neck. Goodness, then, is thought of by the child as exercising control whereby intellectual judgment takes precedence over body impulses.
4. The bad figure generally had some teeth showing, or the lines of the lips were huge and shaded. Frequently, when only a line drawing was made, particularly by younger children, the mouth line went in a downward curve, suggesting unhappiness. In analytic literature it has been observed that aggression is frequently centered about the mouth and teeth. Thus, the child may be expressing, in symbolic terms, the fact that badness means aggressive activity. Teeth appeared in very few of the drawings of good people. Here the lips were often drawn in a kind of cupid's bow, reminiscent of the stereotype for expressing love and affection.
5. The bad person generally wore more articles of clothing than the good

---

[3] K. Machover, *op. cit.,* pp. 56–58.

person. They had more pockets and buttons and more suggestions indicating ties and belts. There was also greater shading in areas representing clothing. Shading is generally suggestive of anxiety. In drawing clothing, the child may be expressing his anxiety in dealing with the concept of badness. He may also, however, be shading those body areas which he associates with "bad" activities. Thus, when the lower portion of the body is shaded, it may be indicative of the anxiety associated with sexual impulses.

6. The figure of the bad person had many more hairy appendages than the figure of the good person. Hair, most generally represented by shading, again is an indication of anxiety. It may also be a displacement of sexual urges. Thus, in drawing hair, the child may be expressing a free-floating anxiety, or he may be expressing an anxiety associated with sexual impulses. Both premises, of course, may be true.

Each child indicated whether his good and bad figures were male or female. Ascribing sex to a figure appeared to be a highly personal conception for each child, depending upon the child's relationship with his parents and his own concept of himself. An equal number of young children considered men bad but women good, or women bad and men good. Some children, of course, drew both figures of the same sex, for both good and bad figures. In adolescence, however, the male figure is most often viewed as the bad figure while the female figure frequently appears as the good person.

In addition to any other interpretations that can be put on them, figure drawings may also represent the child's concept of himself. For instance, a child who feels inadequate may draw a figure in pale yellow, one which all but vanishes into the paper; or perhaps a small lost figure placed either in the center of the paper or unobtrusively hidden in one corner. Robert, for example, made a stick figure alone in the center of a large piece of drawing paper. He was a boy who felt inadequate in an environment which he perceived as threatening. He could not strike out aggressively nor could he withdraw. He was immobilized—he permitted himself to be manipulated by others and thereby merely perpetuated his faulty functioning. Robert's stick figure represents a primitive marionette-like drawing standing all alone. The vastness of the surrounding paper emphasizes his feelings of smallness in terms of the environment. Centering the figure suggests his need to be the focus of his environment.

Dolores, on the other hand, drew a similar figure which she placed, however, in the upper left-hand corner of the page. While her feelings of inadequacy were just as pronounced as those of Robert, she handled these feelings by retreat and withdrawal. By placing the figure as close to the edge of the paper as possible, it appeared as if Dolores herself almost was not there at all.

Just as there are some children like Robert and Dolores who draw small, self-deprecating figures, there are others who cannot contain their figures within the confines of the paper. No matter how large a piece of paper is provided, they ask for additional paper in order to get the extremities placed on the body.

Ethan, for example, used four sheets of newsprint paper 24 inches wide by 30 inches long to complete a whole figure. Ethan was a schizophrenic boy of ten who was overly concerned with his own identity. He was uncertain of himself and his role in the family constellation. He wanted very much to be important, and phantasied himself as more powerful than the rest of the world. His drawings expressed this need to be "big" and significant. As Ethan matured, and developed a more realistic perception of himself, he managed to confine his figures to a 9 inches wide by 12 inches long sheet of paper. His need for self-aggrandizement was still evident, but now represented by theme rather than by size.

Drawings can be an expression of how a child sees himself as well as how he wishes to be. It is difficult to differentiate between these two without knowing more of the child. Freddie, for example, was a nine-year-old boy crippled by polio. He wore braces on both legs and had great difficulty in walking. He drew a boy whose leg was being bitten by a dog. This creative art expression was a reflection of Freddie's physical disability.

In the same way Jordan, a brain-damaged boy, age 8, expressed his own poor muscular co-ordination and lack of equilibrium in a drawing in which one foot was shorter than the other, the arms were unequal, the hands had too many fingers, and the body was grossly asymmetrical.

While this pictorial representation had no basis in reality, since Jordan did not have any obvious physical defect, it was a reflection of the distress which arose from his poor muscular control and his feelings of imbalance. Schizophrenic children often express a similar inner disequilibrium by drawing figures that fly off into space or have disjointed unattached extremities.

Schizophrenic children are also characteristically concerned with space and time. Their artistic expressions often center exclusively about prehistoric life or outer-space phantasies. Martin, a schizophrenic thirteen-year-old boy, was continually occupied in drawing a series of dinosaurs. When he was not drawing them, he was reading about them, writing about them, or making them out of clay, wood, papier-mâché, and cloth which he sewed and stuffed for use as a pillow.

Willie, a nine-year-old schizophrenic boy, used pencil, crayons, and paint, and was as confused in the use of media as he was in himself. He switched from one to the other impulsively and irrationally, using whatever he fell upon regardless of its applicability to the subject.

The expression of inner emotions in art productions can be evaluated not only in terms of content and spatial conception, but also by the use of color. Color is one of the best barometers of a child's emotional life, and can be considered a reflector of emotional interaction. It represents emotional investments in daily experience and indicates a child's willingness and readiness to be spontaneous and to be stimulated by the environment.

The young child, very strongly reactive to environmental stimuli and concerned with the gratification of his own impulses, paints and uses crayons with large, bold strokes and strong colors. He draws as he experiences life—with zest, abandon, and courage. This child may not use color realistically. Although he knows, for example, that a horse is not red, he makes a red horse because, emotionally, red indicates the way he is affected by a horse. He is communicating a feeling rather than a fact.

The young normal child and the young disturbed child use color in much the same way. As they mature, however, a distinction can usually be made between them in terms of their use of color. As the normal child matures, he adds pastel shades and tints, lessening his use of the primary colors. The disturbed child, however, cannot relinquish his use of primary colors, just as he cannot control his emotional responses. His continued use of strong colors indicates his inability to regulate his impulses and drives.

The child who chooses to draw with pencil and rejects the use of color is clearly different from the one who expresses himself in bold colors, and both of these differ from the child who uses muted pastel shades. Bold colors, particularly red, are characteristic of an intense emotional investment in all life experiences and are seen most frequently in the work of very young children. Adolescents, with more emotional maturity, tend to tone down primary colors: the reds become pinks, oranges and yellows; the greens and blues become pale tints. The refusal to use color is seen in both very young and adolescent children who are denying their impulses and avoiding contact with the environment. These children express their depressive and withdrawal tendencies, seek to escape from life, and are afraid of any emotional investment. When the child has complete freedom to explore with no restrictions on his artistic expressions and no imposition of adult standards, the teacher has a rich source for getting to know the child. The teacher must, however, stimulate creativity, particularly with children who have difficulty with spontaneous self-expression.

What about the child who refuses to express himself—who is too inhibited and too threatened by self-revelation to create freely? Here is the child who is mature enough to accept adult standards and is dissatisfied with his representations when they fail to meet these standards. Without reassurance and encouragement, the "artist" in him dies. He cannot express freely, for he cannot experience emotional freedom. He is rooted to his past, and fears the present. A blank piece of paper on which he is asked to draw or write a story seems an immeasurable obstacle. He is holding on rigidly to a tenuous reality which must be constantly redefined by a controlled environment and secured by some restrictions. Restrictions assuage his emotions and afford him less chance to fail in his task. To fail means ridicule with a loss of prestige, and he has not yet learned that failure is a part of learning. His creative expression must start, therefore, with something that does not threaten emotional exposure, but does assure success.

Tracing, a totally uncreative activity, meets both these needs. It is a simple task which is easily construed by the child as an art activity and permits him to participate without releasing his emotions. When enough tracings have been completed successfully and the child feels ready to relinquish this stereotyped activity, he is ready to move on, perhaps to copying, cutting out and recreating pictorial segments or reorganizing the content of his selected picture materials entirely. When he is finally satiated and secure in his success with these activities, he is ready to draw "something out of his own head," as he frequently puts it. Now he can begin to realize the true meaning of creative expression, and his artistic activity can become perceptive and satisfying. Success achieved in creating is carried into other areas, and this child, who can now begin to savor a new fullness in his life, begins to get along in the classroom and make a better adjustment to the entire school program.

Progress is slow, and there are periods of regression and failure, causing the child to take refuge again, perhaps in tracing, but when a particular crisis is passed, creativity begins again. The teacher must understand this behavior, accept it as natural, and continue to support the child in his efforts to meet his emotional needs until he is no longer afraid of his creative artistic expression.

The emotionally disturbed child must be looked at afresh in each new activity and in many situations if the teacher wants to discover more about what "makes him tick." One of the easiest creative arts activities for observing behavior in a group setting is found in music experiences. No matter what the background experiences of the group in musical interests and abilities, every child has a voice. Singing is an extremely gratifying experience which requires no previous training, and permits group participation with the concomitant feeling of belonging. The threat of failure does not exist, and it is not unusual to find that a child who cannot remember that two plus three equals five experiences no difficulty in committing to memory ten or fifteen stanzas of a particular song that he likes. Group singing activities can provide opportunities for individual expression as well, by using a group leader and by encouraging soloists and small singing ensembles. This extension of the singing activity not only offers the group relaxation, but brings extra approval to the special performer from both his peers and the teacher. Much too frequently a child confides that the praise he received for such a contribution was "the only time a teacher ever let me do something I like."

Some children, of course, are so restricted that they hesitate to participate, at first, even in singing. They do, however, often request numbers, indicating that they were enjoying the activity even while playing a passive role. Many children who never contribute voluntarily to any group may become imbued with class spirit. The depressed child can be inspired to sing through his tears and the disruptive bully can release his energies in song. The disturbed child never more closely resembles the normal child than when singing in a group.

The rhythm band is another musical experience that requires no previous training and permits group participation. Children of all ages, including adolescents, can be stimulated to look forward to this activity, which is customarily relegated to the kindergarten, if brushes are used with the drums and popular songs are used as the background. The simple striking instruments of the rhythm band lend themselves well to sublimating aggressive needs in constructive contributions to group enjoyment. Occasionally an overexuberant player thrusts an enthusiastic fist through a drum or tambourine, but fortunately this does not occur very often.

In conjunction with other musical activities, the radio and phonograph play important roles in stimulating creative self-expression. The children are encouraged to engage in associative activities in relation to music. Music is used to stimulate them to write parodies to tunes they like, create new tunes, and draw pictures or model forms to represent the feeling of the music, as well as to respond physically through body movements and dancing. One enthusiastic dancer can spark a whole group, and often almost every child in a room responds to a particular rhythmic recorded selection. This translation of enjoyment into related productive activity is valuable, not only for its momentary satisfaction, but also from a long-range therapeutic point of view. With musically based activities interspersed throughout the school day, sometimes planned and sometimes spontaneous, happy moments are constantly provided to help the disturbed child accept the whole school situation and thereby socialize overt behavior.

Creative artistic expression is by no means limited to art, music, and dance and none of these can be differentiated in terms of value or use. What is said about one can be logically applied to all, and the advantages of these expressions are pertinent to all other related areas. Finger painting, clay modeling, wood whittling, and crafts projects permit the child to respond to the feel of the materials as well as to the sight of what he is creating. This response to "feel" reveals additional clues to personality. Does he enjoy messing with finger paints? Does he carefully construct a delicate ceramic object or does he pound his clay figure into a satisfyingly shapeless mass? Is his papier-mâché puppet given life and reality by a name and the attribution of human characteristics? Does he relax most in the physical activity of the woodworking shop and obtain his release from tension through satisfaction in construction? One almost cannot exhaust all the possibilities inherent in the daily school lives of these children for the unfolding of artistic creative expression, and their use for the release of pent-up emotions. Although not all activities are equally projective in nature, and each may represent only one small momentary phase of a total personality pattern, when responses in several areas are studied, trends begin to take shape and changes begin to take on significance.

SUMMARY

The creative arts offer the maladjusted child ways to externalize his emotions and make satisfactory contact with the environment. It offers the former failure and recalcitrant some nonacademic, conflict-free areas of activity directed toward realistic individual goals, within which he can grow in confidence and obtain a goodly measure of success. Praise and approval of desirable behavior now net him greater satisfactions than his former aggressive or withdrawal patterns. He is learning how to adjust and how to be happy.

Chapter XI

The Academic Curriculum

In a school for disturbed children where each child is practically a class by himself, it is difficult to speak in terms of an academic curriculum for a group. Instead, of necessity, the teacher must think in terms of the individual child and how a curriculum can best meet this child's needs. The most basic among these needs, of course, is a need for an effective reading program.

Regardless of the various types of children described as problems, the majority suffer from some degree of retardation in reading. Emotional maladjustment can cause academic retardation, and academic retardation can contribute considerably to a child's emotional problems. When one considers the fact that children spend the major portion of their waking day in school, the interrelationship between reading retardation and emotional problems is apparent.

The importance of a reading disability cannot be underestimated, for a reading disability is a disability in almost every area of learning. The child who has a reading disability is usually below grade level in spelling, writing, social studies, and so on. Thus a reading disability can cause complete failure in school, and surely the child who is failing in all academic areas must suffer emotionally.

The overwhelming importance of reading failure and its relationship to other areas necessitates a search for effective methodology in the teaching of remedial reading. What methods can be devised to assure even a small measure of success in teaching a child to read—a child who in spite of years of schooling has failed to learn? The first step is to get the child to admit that he has difficulty with reading. Often the child is so discouraged with his own lack of achievement that to get him to admit he needs help is a major success for the teacher. It takes a great deal of time before the child is able to make this kind of admission. The time in building a working relationship between pupil and teacher is well spent, however, for without a trusting relationship, a relationship in which the child asks for help and the teacher offers it, remediation cannot be effective. In fact, remedial reading offered when the child is still resistive can only lead to further interpersonal difficulties between teacher and pupil, and to greater emotional conflict for the child.

In starting reading, it is usually not feasible for the child to use the materials with which he has formerly failed. A child who has not succeeded with the usual textbooks found in the schoolrooms throughout the country, is not ready to pick up these selfsame books and start again. The book is associated in the child's mind with failure and the resultant emotional distress that accompanies failure. Furthermore, while these books are of interest to the great majority of school children, they do not maintain an interest for the disturbed child who cannot center his thought processes on the realistic situations often portrayed in the texts. Early-grade readers most often emphasize the life of a child in the home and community. Family life, however, is frequently a major source of conflict to the disturbed child. He usually does not have good family relationships; he is too attached to his mother or too antagonistic; his feelings toward his father are fraught with resentment toward authority; and he has difficulties with sibling relationships. How then can he concentrate upon readers centered on family life, readers often illustrated with pictures of well-dressed, happy-looking children who live under the most ideal conditions? The disturbed child who does not get along with his family, and who is not happy, obviously will not read such texts. Rather, this kind of reading material heightens his emotional conflicts and reinforces his resistance to reading.

Because all children have a vivid sense of phantasy, disturbed children in particular, it is best to introduce them to reading with stories like "The Little Red Hen," "The Gingerbread Boy," or "The Country Mouse and the City Mouse." In other words, reading materials consisting of fairy tales, fables, and other forms of phantasy have proven to be of great value in the introduction of reading. Two factors may be largely responsible for the success of this kind of story. First, these stories are real stories, containing the best elements of drama, excitement, and even mystery. They build up to intensive climaxes; their resolutions are emotionally satisfying. This is not so with the modern-day readers, which stress everyday experiential living, but which are not nearly as interesting or as provocative. Second, and perhaps more important, is that the child can accept any fantastic story at face value. That is, fairy tales permit the use of conflict situations which the child might ordinarily reject because of their proximity to reality. Fairy tales and myths, however, disguise the obvious realistic situations which children might otherwise find emotionally threatening. Thus a child can identify with the Gingerbread Boy running away from the old woman without experiencing the guilt he might feel if he were to read about a little boy running away from his mother. With the fantastic world of folk legend, any child accepts the story, is entertained by the situation, and infers from it those aspects which apply to him. When children empathize with the animal hero of a story and make identifications, they gain some insight into their own behavior patterns and emotions and develop a rationale for the behavior of others. Certainly the story of the three little kittens who lost their mittens would not be as terrifying to a child as the story of a real little boy who was punished by his mother for losing something. A child can more easily accept a story with a punishment theme, and accept all the emotional concomitants attached to it, if the situation is once removed from reality. In this way he can accept the story, discuss it, and perhaps benefit from it, knowing all the time that it is not really true. The knowledge that a story is "make-believe" offers emotional release and catharsis without being traumatic and disturbing.

The best means of obtaining reading materials which are emotionally satisfying to the child without disturbing him are by procuring those materials from the children themselves. The technique of using the child's own compositions for reading is, of course, not new. Every teacher of reading uses experiential charts in which the child tells about his trip to the zoo, or what the class did the preceding day. Children love to read the words they have spoken, but usually these words are centered on reality situations. The disturbed child, however, sees reality differently. He may not want to write about a birthday party he attended, particularly if this social experience was an unhappy one for him. But he would like to write about something he made up from his own imagination. His experiential background is replete with phantasy, for phantasy is more real to him than the real world. It is this phantasy material which can be used most effectively in teaching him how to read. A child tells his story, the teacher types or prints it for him, the child illustrates it, and then the booklet is bound. The child then has his own "phantasy booklet," which becomes his own reader. Sometimes the procedure may be reversed, with the child drawing the story before the teacher puts it into print.

Reading thus becomes a most satisfying activity, providing the child with the opportunity to express his own interests and to have these interests accepted by the teacher. For example, the following sentences were dictated by a ten-year-old, one for each page of a four-page booklet in which he had drawn pictures representing the story he was planning to learn to read:

1. This is Superman who will scare away the wolves from the house.
2. Superman is flying over the people and the houses.
3. Superman is shooting electricity and lightning into the water.
4. Superman is a good guy and so is Dracula, Frankenstein, and blood-suckers. They are all good to me. The end.

When the teacher accepts any and all such story material regardless of its unreality, as if it were common experience, the child, perhaps for the first time in his life, can feel that he is an accepted part of a learning group. He is then encouraged to pursue his studies further. When the program of phantasy reading is carried to its logical conclusion, the child soon develops a large enough reading sight vocabulary to permit him to relinquish his own phantasy material as a source of learning in favor of available readers. At this point, the child feels that he can learn to read, and the commercial readers are no longer a threat to him. He can accept the experiences of the other children, his own phantasy world giving way to the more accepted patterns of reality.

What has the teacher done in accepting stories from the child? In essence, in accepting the child's stories without commenting that they are foolish or silly, the teacher has accepted the child. Again, one finds that need-acceptance therapy is most effective. The child feels that the teacher likes him because the stories, no matter how weird, have not been censured. The child also feels that perhaps he is not so very different after all, if his stories are accepted without reference to their absurdity. For the first time in his life, the child may feel that he is like other children, and feeling this way, he attempts more and more to be like them. He no longer needs his own phantasy. Because he has been given free rein in expressing even the most unacceptable ideas, the ideas themselves and the emotions underlying them are no longer disturbing to him. He has expressed his phantasy and now he is willing to let it go.

The adolescent who is somewhat inhibited artistically, and not so free in his art productions as the young child, is not able to utilize phantasy material in art expression. He can, however, be introduced to reading with a kind of unique word list. He may be asked, for instance, "If you could learn only five or six words in your whole life, which words would you want to learn most of all?" The reading can then be started with this word list. The words any one child chooses are frequently much more difficult than any the teacher would ordinarily choose. Sometimes these word lists appear to have no reasonable order except in the mind of the child. For instance, this word list was prepared by a fifteen-year old boy: "Wolfman, zombie, wife, weight-lifting, and Atlas." A thirteen-year old said: "Grandmother, Count of Monte Cristo, cat, and chocolate." A sixteen-year old girl said: "Actress, hypochondriac, antidisestablishmentarianism, and turquoise."

Amazingly, the child who could not seem to remember "up, up, up" and "down, down, down" from the basic primers, managed to learn and retain the words of his own choosing. This kind of list can be increased daily, and when enough words are learned, the adolescent can be encouraged to attempt a phantasy booklet with the words he already knows.

Using the same personal reader type of format as the phantasy booklets, the tape recorder may be added to the program as a further incentive toward learning to read. Following the pattern of the commercial record albums, the child can dictate his original story to the teacher, who types three or four sentences on a page. The child invents a sound which means "turn the page." The story is then read into the microphone and after that—for drill—the child listens to his own voice telling the story, while he follows it on the typed pages. The fascination of this activity seems to be endless, and both children and adolescents appear never to tire of hearing themselves. Learning to read in this way can really be painless.

Using songs can be another "painless" way of learning to read. With young children a special type of song is used—action songs.[1] Action songs help children to express normal, natural needs in a socially acceptable manner. Children like to act with their bodies, to sway their hips, to reach up with their hands, to whirl their heads. Action songs, providing these movement experiences, can be used with reading. After the children learn the words of a song in association with action, they learn the words from the written page. The words are duplicated on separate sheets of paper and the child reads them while he sings. In addition, to vary the procedure and to force attention onto the words, the child is provided with a magnet and a metal bar. The child holds the magnet under the paper, moving it from word to word; the little bar, resting on top of the paper, follows the magnet. The activity becomes similar to the bouncing ball type of singing done in movie theaters. Adolescents particularly like this activity. With them, however, popular songs may be used.

This kind of reading is purposeful even when the purpose is unknown to the child. It is entertaining, done in a social situation, and focuses the child's attention upon words without his being aware that he is

---

[1] See E. Rothman and P. Berkowitz, "Let's Sing a Little Action" (New York: Lawson-Gould Music Publishers, 1955).

reading. Under these conditions, the attention span of even the most distractible child can be extended, and learning can take place without stress or pressure.

Another device which is of interest to the disturbed child, helping him to maintain attention and participate with enthusiasm, is a battery-operated quiz-game type of reading drill. This consists of a series of reading cards superimposed upon the usual commercial quiz boards having two leads and a red light. The cards can be teacher-made, specifically designed to assist in sound discrimination and word identification. Special cards may be allotted for word recognition, picture matching, vowel discrimination, initial consonant recognition, consonant blends, and so on. The following example is a card for consonant blends. The teacher or another child says the blend and the child picks out the sound with one wire. On the other side of the card, he matches the blend. When the correct match is made, a red light goes on.

MATCHING

sp	br	kl	ch	sp	cl
cr	sh	cl	br	th	cr
pl	th	ch	sh	pl	kl

Several variations, of course, can be played. The teacher and children can use their ingenuity to devise different rules of playing. This game has real value because it holds the interest of almost every child who attempts to work with it. The child is intrigued by the mechanics of the game and delights in the red light which indicates a correct choice of response.

No one method will work with all children, and regardless of method there are those children who seem not to be able to learn. Even those who are learning seem at times to backslide and give little indication of the amount of effort which has been expended in order to help them. However, in spite of the failures and inadequacies in both knowledge and methodology, many children who seem previously to have had no ability to learn to read can actually be taught and can improve in their skill. With enough patience and a tremendous capacity for accepting uneven progress along with successes, one can take a sanguine view of the progress which can be made in the teaching of reading.

Spelling, as we know, is closely related to skill in reading. For success in spelling, it has been found that it is necessary to have a large reading vocabulary and to be able to remember and reproduce letters correctly. While some children may have the reading vocabulary necessary for spelling, they nevertheless have difficulty in perceiving and reproducing letters. Such children generally are those whose diagnosis includes an organic disturbance.

When this type of child learns to write a single manuscript letter, the problem of the connection of letters in cursive writing exists. He finds it difficult to make connecting lines. Thus, he learns how to write *m* alone but he cannot learn *ms* or *ma*. In teaching, therefore, when the letters must be presented with the connecting line between them, the child should write these on a clay board as well as on paper with a pencil. Cursive writing, approached in this way, becomes much less of a problem. Most children, when learning cursive writing in school, start with the simple vertical lines such as *i* and *t*. These are the most difficult letters for the child with an organic abnormality, who finds it impossible, at first, to make a vertical line and then retrace the *same* line, going in a different direction. Thus, in teaching cursive writing, these special difficulties must be kept in mind, so that letters like *i* and *t* are taught after letters like *e, l, m,* and *n* have been mastered.

The most important academic learning area other than the language arts is arithmetic. While the disturbed child has difficulty with arithmetic in the understanding of concepts and in the solving of problems, he generally has acquired some proficiency in the practical use of numbers. Children very early learn practical everyday use of money. While they may not understand the concept of a computation, they frequently have memorized a correct response. A child, therefore, who may not understand that division results in a smaller number while multiplication results in a larger number, can nevertheless multiply and divide with accuracy. The discrepancy, therefore, between arithmetic functioning and intellectual ability is usually not as great as the discrepancy between reading and intellectual ability. In the teaching of arithmetic, the emphasis must, therefore, be placed on the development of concepts. Since the basic combinations are largely familiar to the child, there is no need to use contrived phantasy materials. Concept development can be based upon experiential classroom activities.

The learning of arithmetic skills, like the learning of reading, depends on a unique presentation of materials directed specifically toward the development of concepts. Instead of rote memorization of combinations, the concept of two plus three, for example, is best presented through the use of group objects—blocks, sticks, balloons, lollipops, etc. The teacher may say, "Take a group of two, add a group of three." The child gets the answer by beginning with the concept of two as a group and adding three objects as a group, to get an answer of five which may now be visualized as a total of groups. If the teacher says, "Add two and three," the concept of a group may be lost if the child merely counts. The concept of adding a group would then not be present and the child would be manipulating discrete forms rather than abstracting a concept. The visual presentation of arithmetic materials may not be enough, however. The child must not only handle the materials, but, if possible, they should offer resistance so that learning can be reinforced by motor activity. For instance, the stick groups should have to be placed into a peg board or the blocks should have to be placed in a form board. In addition, the child could write the combination in clay, finger paints, with pen and ink, in oils, on textured paper, with a typewriter, etc., in fact, using any media which require concentration and motor movement and offer a certain amount of inherent resistance and difficulty. When this kind of motor reinforcement procedure is repeated often enough, the child will be able to understand the concept.

If a child's increase in the understanding of arithmetical concepts and number relationships is concomitant with an increase in reading ability, success in problem solving follows naturally. Academic emphasis in the areas of reading and concept development in arithmetic forms a basis for success in total school achievement. Proficiency in these areas is necessary for successful participation in all academic subjects.

In summary, the three R's, reading, writing, and arithmetic, form the basic academic curriculum for the disturbed child. While disturbed children may be stimulated by science experiments and interested in social studies units, and while they can contribute to these activities in a nonacademic, peripheral way, they cannot participate meaningfully in organized, sequentially planned lessons unless they have the basic academic skills. Until such skills are acquired, therefore, the social studies and science curriculum, of necessity, must be limited to isolated experiences and short, discrete units.

Chapter XII

Transcript of a Classroom Session

The material presented in this chapter was obtained in a classroom located in a psychiatric hospital. It consists of the actual proceedings recorded during a morning session in a class for disturbed boys. The children were unaware that the recording was being taken and were, therefore, free and spontaneous in their behavior. The three-hour transcript is obviously much too extensive to present here in its entirety. The accounts which follow, therefore, are those selected sections which were most significant in terms of understanding the children, as well as those which demonstrated some of the practices described here previously. The comments between sections attempt to point out some of this significant material. A brief description of the class follows:

BERT, age nine, was diagnosed as a schizophrenic child. He was placed in the hospital because of severe cigarette burns which he had inflicted upon his arms. His school history was one of almost complete failure. He read on a first-grade level. His arithmetic skill was on a second-grade level. He had been in constant difficulty in the public schools he attended, generally putting himself into positions whereby the abuse of others would be heaped upon him. He constantly tattled on the other children. In the hospital school, his behavior was almost euphoric. He constantly talked of his happiness. He was engaged in endless crafts activities, particularly in braiding seemingly millions of yards of rope, with increasing zest for each yard.

HARVEY, age eleven, was referred to the hospital for diagnosis after excessive truanting from the public schools and after having been found aimlessly wandering around the waterfront. In both reading and arithmetic he was on a third-grade level. In the community, Harvey had engaged in petty thefts and had been in conflict with the law. In the hospital school he was quietly impulsive and destructive. He destroyed other children's work and cut up books and papers with a pair of scissors which seemed to be always ready for action in his hand. Harvey was diagnosed as a primary behavior problem.

JAY, nine years of age, had come to the hospital because of his bizarre behavior in the public school. He got involved in frequent fights and spoke quite comfortably with a man who lived inside of him. He was a complete nonreader and had no arithmetic concepts. In the hospital, his behavior was erratic, bizarre, and impulsive. He alternated between periods of extreme aggression and periods of passivity. He was diagnosed as schizophrenic.

RODNEY, age ten, was a schizophrenic boy who was referred for psychiatric diagnosis by the convalescent home in which he had proved too difficult to manage. His ability to read phonetically was on grade level. His vocabulary was also on grade level. His comprehension, however, was second grade. He was hyperactive, and highly imaginative in play. His phantasy centered upon living in a "fox hole," the label he gave to his usual seat underneath a bench or table. In addition to Rodney, the "fox hole" was occupied by an alarm clock, a blanket, a little Christmas tree, books, pencils, jar covers, bits of colored paper and other assorted treasures.

RICKY, age nine, a schizophrenic boy, was admitted to the hospital after running away from home. He would not read or do arithmetic. In the hospital he was passive and compliant. He liked to dress up in girls' clothing and pretend he was a girl. He drew pictures that were obscene and seemed preoccupied with sexual concerns.

HERBERT, age twelve, came to the hospital after excessive truanting and overt misbehavior in school. He was a nonreader, but his arithmetic skill was on a fifth-grade level. He was destructive, impulsive, and aggressive in school. He was diagnosed as a primary behavior problem.

CLAUDE was twelve years of age when he was admitted to the hospital. He had been a problem at home and at school, running away from both at frequent intervals. He read on a third-grade level but had no skill in arithmetic except with practical money affairs. In the hospital school he was liked by everyone. He was polite, co-operative, and a wonderfully charming liar. He, too, was diagnosed as schizophrenic.

At nine o'clock in the morning, the hospital attendant ushered the children into the room.

BERT (Diving to the floor, kissing it and squealing): Oh-h-h, I'm so glad to be in school. (Getting up from floor) Teach, where's my rope?

HERBERT: Out of my way, boy! Move!

TEACHER: Good morning, Bert. Good morning, Harvey. (Harvey goes to corner of room, picking up scissors on way.) Good morning, Jay. Good morning, Herbert. Good morning, Claude.

RICKY: Teacher, I'm going to paint.

TEACHER: That's fine. Good morning, Ricky.

JAY: Where's my lanyard?

RICKY: Where are the paints, teacher?

JAY: I want my lanyard.

TEACHER: Where they always are, Ricky, on the easel.

HERBERT: Stupid question—stupid answer.

JAY: Where's my lanyard?

HERBERT: F—— your lanyard.

RICKY: There's no pink, teacher!

JAY: I want my lanyard—open the desk, teach.

TEACHER: You have to make pink yourself. Here's your rope, Bert.

RICKY: Show me how. (Teacher goes over to Ricky to help him mix paint.)

JAY: I put my lanyard in your drawer.

TEACHER: Now, just a minute, Jay. I'll get it for you in a moment. Wait till I mix the pink for Ricky. What are you going to do, Claude?

JAY: I don't want to wait. Everybody gets things first.

HERBERT: Want me to make him shut up, teach?

TEACHER (Getting paper from closet): I'll be with you in a moment, Jay. When I need your help, Herbert, I'll ask for it.

JAY: You always say that—wait, wait, what do you think I am, a waiter?

RICKY: Waiter, potater—you got a big potater—I'm gonna paint your prick potater.

RODNEY: I'm late, teacher, I had to see my doctor.

CLAUDE: Make him keep still. Some kids talk too much. Think they are big—they are small.

TEACHER: Good morning, Rodney. What would you like to do today?

BERT: That's right, Claude. Smarty pants, smarty pants—Ricky is a smarty pants.

RODNEY: I'm going into my fox hole to read my workbook. Give me a pencil.

RICKY: You're a smarty pants, you're a farty pants, fart in your pants.

CLAUDE: Words, words, words, words, words, words, words.

HERBERT: Hey teach—you gonna let these kids talk like that?

JAY (Screaming): Teacher, I'm waiting.

HERBERT: Hey teach—you a real teacher? How come you let them talk like that?

TEACHER: I'll be right with you, Jay.

HERBERT: Dirty words. Shit! I can't stand them.

JAY: I'm waiting—I'm waiting.

HERBERT: You heard her, you bastard. She said she'd be with you.

BERT: Look at my rope. Isn't it beautiful, teacher?

TEACHER: It is magnificent. (Pause) Herbert, are you finishing that lovely mural you started?

JAY: You see that—she helps everyone and not me.

TEACHER: I'll be with you in a minute, Jay.

HERBERT: Hey teacher—let him wait—I need more water.

TEACHER: It looks beautiful. Take the pitcher from my desk and fill it with water from the sink.

RODNEY: Come and see me in my fox hole.

TEACHER: Yes, I will, Rodney. I might even bring a friend with me. (The teacher finished helping Ricky mix paints and went to Jay. Rodney crawled back into his corner between the woodworking bench and the wall.) All right, Jay. Now, let's see what you would like.

RICKY: What he'd like is a girl friend.

HARVEY: I'd like a gun.

JAY: I told you, my lanyard. I put it in your drawer.

TEACHER: Well, let's look. (Pause) It's not here now. Are you sure you put it here?

JAY: I put it right there in the drawer.

TEACHER: I'm sorry, Jay. It's not here now. You should have given it to me.

JAY: Somebody stole it.

BERT: You stole it yourself.

TEACHER: Nobody stole it. It must be misplaced.

CLAUDE: Stolen? Misplaced? Who would steal it? Why would anyone steal it? Just go to the closet—there's lots of it there—just take it from the closet.

JAY: Somebody stole it.

HERBERT (Re-entering the room): You calling me a crook?

BERT: Yeah, he's calling you a crook.

CLAUDE: Just take it from the closet.

TEACHER: As a matter of fact, Jay, I just remembered. I took that lanyard home. It was so beautiful and I needed it for my key. I hope you don't mind, but I needed it so badly, I just might have lost my key. How about making me another now? I need one for my school key, too.

JAY: You want the same diamond stitch, you Sunday teacher?

TEACHER: What do you mean—Sunday teacher?

JAY: You're not working. What kind of stitch do you want?

TEACHER: Surprise me, Jay. I know it will be lovely. What are you doing, Claude?

CLAUDE: Thank God that's settled. Talk, talk, talk. Are you ready? I'm wating to help you with the movie machine.

TEACHER: Oh, that's sweet, Claude. I do need your help, but that's not till eleven o'clock. Let's plan what we're going to do until then. You go to the blackboard.

By this time, the teacher had provided a constructive activity for each child except Harvey, who was sitting in the far corner of the room methodically destroying a large box of his crayons. A mound of colored shavings and cuttings had appeared at the foot of his chair. While the teacher was aware of this behavior, she was also aware that this behavior was an indication of improvement. The very fact that he was destroying his own property and not the work of others meant that he had reached the point where he could be contained within the classroom without disrupting the structure of the group. She chose to treat him with intelligent neglect and permit him to work out his aggressions at this moment for himself.

It is obvious from the conversation that took place that many of the others had problems in controlling aggression, both in terms of obscene language and overt behavior. Herbert was quick to seize upon several situations which could have led to a fight, and each of which Bert was happy to encourage. The teacher averted the overt aggression in one case by assuming the blame for the disappearance of the lanyard which actually had been her responsibility. She remembered that it had been left out overnight and realized that it had probably been thrown away. Knowing that Jay would interpret this as a rejection she assumed a subservient role and asked him for his help. This role not only served Jay by meeting his need for status, but it also helped Herbert by saving him from his own impulsive aggression.

At this point, the picture of the classroom was one of varying degrees of activity and inactivity. Claude was obviously just waiting for eleven o'clock. Harvey was destroying his own materials. Ricky was painting at the easel, while Herbert was painting a mural on the board. Rodney was reading under a desk and Jay was starting a lanyard. Using Claude's reference to the audio-visual program for which the class was scheduled, the teacher was able to hold a group discussion for a very short period of time during which each child outlined his own activities and goals for the day and the class as a whole considered the group activities which they were going to join. Starting with an orientation of day and time, the teacher opened the discussion by asking what day and date it was, and had each child repeat it. Claude then wrote the day, date, and plans for the day on the board for all to read. Even while they were planning together, each child was busy with his own project.

To have attempted a group discussion without first involving each child in an individual project would have invited disaster. The group discussion, however, was profitable in that each child was learning how to contribute to a group even though he was individually occupied.

The teacher had Claude put the plans on the board as they were evolved by the pupils, and asked certain children to read them. Rodney peeked out of his fox hole to contribute to the general discussion. As this group discussion ended, the children turned their attention back to their own interests.

TEACHER: Claude, here is your arithmetic paper. As soon as you finish it you can set up the projector. Rodney, how about showing me your work? Let's see how far you've gotten.

RODNEY: No, you come here to my fox hole.

TEACHER: I'm too big and it's too dark down there to read.

RODNEY: It's not dark—foxes can see good here.

TEACHER: Suppose I meet you halfway—right at Ricky's desk.

RICKY: Don't touch anything on that desk.

TEACHER: We'll be very careful.

HERBERT: Fussy faggot. Got nothin' on his old desk.

RICKY (Low mutter): Black bitch.

TEACHER: Rodney, let's go over your work. (Teacher and Rodney stay at Ricky's desk and for about ten minutes they go over the reading lesson which was planned for Rodney. There was relative quiet in the room during this time and each child seemed absorbed in his own project.) That was wonderful. It was so good I have a surprise for you. You'll have to come all the way to my desk for it.

RODNEY: What is it? (Teacher took from underneath a desk an old fox scarf which had a head and tail.)

TEACHER: This is a fox for your fox hole.

CLAUDE: A fox? A real fox? Is it a real fox?

HERBERT: Dumb bastard.

RODNEY: Gee, thanks—I'm going to take him home when I leave.

JAY: I'll make a lanyard for your fox if you want me to, Rodney.

BERT: I'll make him a rope.

RICKY: I'll sew him a coat.

HERBERT: I'll walk him for you.

HARVEY (Relinquishing his scissors for the first time): I'll go with you.

TEACHER: No, boys, he had a long trip in this morning. He's too tired to walk just now.

BERT: Let's read him a story.

HERBERT: Let's not.

TEACHER: That's a splendid idea. What story shall we read?

RODNEY (Pointing to the fox): He wants "Little Red Riding Hood."

TEACHER: Harvey, would you get the book from the story shelf, please, while we all gather around the table to hear the story?

HERBERT (As he draws his chair up to the table): That's sissy stuff!

CLAUDE: Is it eleven o'clock?

TEACHER: Not yet, dear. Do you want to listen to this story?

CLAUDE: I'll finish my examples and set up the machine.

(Teacher reads to the group.)

It is apparent that the teacher was aware of the work Rodney was doing and was fully prepared to work with him individually. It is also apparent that Rodney resisted the lesson. The teacher had no need to maintain prestige in front of the group and therefore she did not insist that he obey her. Instead, she met him on his own terms in a game-like approach and made it easy for him to conform by giving him an opportunity to meet her halfway. She also ignored Ricky's and Herbert's language, aware that chastising them would only create a conflict situation.

The teacher found it expedient to enter Rodney's phantasy life and thereby help him to express his bizarre ideation. By accepting his phantasies herself, she was helping him toward eventually relinquishing his phantasy for reality. It is clear that the other children saw no incongruity in the teacher's participation in this unreality. They all seemed to play along with it, using it for their own purposes, but knowing all the time that it was actually phantasy.

Herbert clearly attempted to separate Rodney from his fox by playing along with this make-believe, using it to veil his overt aggressive behavior. The teacher was sensitive to Herbert's needs and stepped in, once again, alleviating the possibility of conflict by diverting him with an apparently reasonable explanation.

Claude, whose goal was eleven o'clock and the machine he was going to operate, applied himself diligently to the arithmetic the teacher had prepared for him, undaunted by the fox, the fox hole and the story being read to the class. Claude was obsessed with movie projectors. He was not concerned with the film and its content, but rather with the mechanics of a motion picture machine. This interest seemed to be the prime motivating force for all his overt behavior.

After the teacher finished reading the story, the following ensued:

TEACHER: Why did you want this story, Rodney?
RODNEY: Because it's got a wolf and if we act out the story the fox can play the part of the wolf.
TEACHER: Who would you be, Rodney, if we acted it out?
RODNEY: I'd be the wolf's brother and help him fight the woodsman.
HERBERT: I'd be the woodsman and I'd chop your head off.
RICKY: Not mine, 'cause I'd be Little Red Riding Hood.
JAY: No, I'd be Little Red Riding Hood.
HERBERT: You fat f——. You're too fat.
HARVEY: I'll be the grandmother.
TEACHER: Claude, what about you?
CLAUDE: Is it eleven o'clock yet?
TEACHER: No, dear. It's 10:30 now.
CLAUDE: I think I'll get the machine.
TEACHER: Let me have your arithmetic work. We will go over it together right after lunch.
BERT: We going to act it out?
HERBERT: Shut up!

JAY: Shut down!

BERT: I want to play the mouse in "Cinderella."

RODNEY: You can't be the mouse. The fox has to be the mouse.

TEACHER: Suppose you could be a character in any story you know. Who would you want to be? One at a time.

BERT: I want to be Supermouse.

HERBERT: I want to be Robin Hood.

RODNEY: I'd like to be a fox and live in the woods with Robin Hood and Little John.

RICKY: Little John is a little bathroom.

JAY: You ill-brained child.

RICKY: You pill monster.

JAY: I'm not a pill monster.

HERBERT: You're a faggot!

TEACHER: Harvey, what would you like to be?

HARVEY: Perry Mason. I see him on TV every week.

JAY: Teacher, can I make my pot holder now?

TEACHER: Let me hold your lanyard and you can get the loops from the closet.

RICKY: Oh-h-h, I want to make one too.

TEACHER: How about reading first, Ricky? Then you can make a pot holder.

RICKY: All right. Let me get my loops to hold.

TEACHER: I have your book right here on my desk. Herbert, would you like to bring your book up also? You can read with us.

HERBERT: I have to go to the bathroom.

BERT: I want to read, teacher. I can read that book too.

TEACHER: Fine, bring the clay board and you can write the words in clay.

BERT: And my stick for the clay.

TEACHER: Harvey, you are so careful when you help me—would you please water the plants? They look very thirsty.

HERBERT: I want to type my new words on the typewriter.

TEACHER: When you come back from the bathroom.

HERBERT: I don't have to go. I want to type.

TEACHER: Fine. Here is your word list.

At this point, the group again returned into individualized activity. Each child was engaged in an activity—academic or nonacademic. Each activity, moreover, was the one the child selected for himself during the planning period. Each child appeared happy in what he was doing, and the over-all tenor of the class appeared to be friendly and busy.

During the entire discussion about Red Riding Hood, the teacher was providing the children with an opportunity for emotional expression. Her acceptance of the role each child wanted to play was in essence an acceptance of the child himself. The children clearly felt free to express themselves without fear of censure. This was therefore a cathartic and supportive experience for them. The differences between the children were clearly defined in the choice of masculine or feminine roles. Ricky and Jay gave evidence of female identification. Herbert chose a completely masculine role, indicating that he made a masculine identification. Bert and Rodney indicated a more primitive level of functioning in that they identified with nonhumans. Harvey evidenced some confusion in identification alternating between assuming the masculine and feminine roles. Claude, still removed from the group, was cleaning the lens and oiling the projector.

The discussion had petered out in quite a natural manner and the children returned to selected, planned, individual activities. Jay, for instance, followed the assignments he had selected for himself that day. Ricky and Claude, however, needed help in keeping to their goals. The teacher assisted them unobtrusively, always keeping the children interested in what they were doing. With Harvey, however, the teacher's prime concern was keeping him busy with socially acceptable experiences which were satisfying to him and which were not disruptive to the group. Harvey was still at the stage of testing his own acceptability, and he was not emotionally ready for more structured activity.

After this period of individual activity, the audio-visual program was scheduled to start and the classroom procedure was as follows:

TEACHER: Claude, it's eleven o'clock now—are you all set?

CLAUDE: All ready to go. I've been all ready all day. I'm always all ready.

TEACHER: Let's put everything away now and set up the chairs.

CLAUDE: Just bring the chairs over—I'll set them up. Let me through—I've got to pull down the shades—is everyone set? Ready? Oh, put out the lights—it's eleven o'clock.

TEACHER: Wait just a minute, Claude. First let us talk a little. Who remembers the name of the film—we wrote it on the blackboard when we made our plans for today.

BERT: "Party Lines."

TEACHER: Who can tell us what the film is about?

JAY: About parties?

BERT: Whose party? A Christmas party.

RICKY: It's about pencil lines.

BERT: I made a rope on a pencil once—it was a horse rein.

HERBERT: I remember, teach—it's about telephones.

CLAUDE: I saw it before when I showed it to the other class—it takes twenty minutes.

TEACHER: Tell us what it is about.

CLAUDE: What's it about—what do you mean what's it about?

TEACHER: Well, what does the story tell us?

CLAUDE: What does it tell? the story? You get me all mixed up.

TEACHER: Well, as Herbert told us, the film is about telephones. Now what is a party line?

CLAUDE: A party line? What's a party line?

HARVEY: It's like someone else can hear what you say when you talk.

TEACHER: That's true—what else can you tell us about a party line?

HERBERT: They got the same telephone in another house you don't know. When we moved into the project the dames was always gab-gab-gab on my phone—all day. I cussed them and my father cussed them and they never did shut up.

BERT: Was it their phone or your phone?

HERBERT: It was my goddamn phone.

JAY: I wouldn't let anybody talk on my phone. What right do they have to come in your house anyway?

RICKY: Yeah—what right? Some people have some nerve!

TEACHER: A party line means that two phones in two different homes are connected to the same trunk line. The film will explain exactly how a party line works and will help us understand why we must use the party line phone with consideration for others. Claude, you can start the film now.

CLAUDE: Everyone sit down—stop talking—look at the screen—turn off the lights, teach.

At the conclusion of the film, Claude busied himself rewinding the film and dismantling the machine for its return to the closet. With the rest of the group, the teacher reviewed the material presented in the film. The discussion centered upon the behavior of the marionettes in the story. The film depicted emergency situations which require the immediate use of a phone to obtain assistance and the proper use of the telephone in daily living.

JAY: I like to talk on the telephone. It's fun.

BERT: I talked long distance once and it sounded like it was in the next room.

HERBERT: That's the way it's supposed to sound when you have a good connection.

TEACHER: Right. What else did we learn from the film?

HARVEY: Be polite and when you get the wrong number you say, "Excuse me."

HERBERT: It's better if you dial the right number first.

BERT: And when there's a fire you have to get off the phone.

TEACHER: What happened in the movie when someone did not get off the phone for an emergency?

RICKY: The house burned down because someone wouldn't get off the line and let the men call the fire department.

TEACHER: Exactly. What lesson did we learn?

BERT: Don't talk a long time, and let someone else use it.

JAY: Can you call God on the telephone?

CLAUDE: Call God on the telephone? You mean God? God up in heaven?

BERT: I want to call Santa Claus 'cause I have to tell him that I'm a little Jewish boy and I don't have a Christmas tree in my house but if he comes anyway to bring me a present I'll leave a piece of chaleh with honey on the mantelpiece for him.

HERBERT: Get that—he still believes in Santa Claus!

RICKY: Santa Claus wouldn't come to Jay. He is always taking things. You know those clips you lost? Jay took them.

JAY: I did not! Search me, teach.

RICKY: He's got them in his pockets.

CLAUDE: Pockets? Do we have a film about pockets?

BERT: You won't find anything, teacher—his outside pockets are empty.

TEACHER: What do you mean, "his outside pockets"?

BERT: He wears two pairs of pants—a pair for searching on top and a pair for stealing underneath.

TEACHER: Well, that's very clever, Jay. We'll talk about the clips later.

JAY: I didn't steal them, teacher, I found them and I was just going to give them to you.

TEACHER: Jay, if my telephone number is BAyville 6-1250 and you want to call me, how would you dial this number?

JAY: You just do the first two—the B and the A—and then you do all the numbers after that.

TEACHER: That's right. I have some telephones here. Let's practice dialing numbers.

As a final reinforcement, this audio-visual session culminated in an opportunity for each child to use a demonstration two-way telephone set. With this activity, the morning session ended and the children were escorted to lunch by a hospital attendant.

INDEX

Index